THE SYNTHESIS
OF SELF

VOLUME 1
THE I OF CONSCIOUSNESS
Development from Birth to Maturity

THE SYNTHESIS OF SELF
Roy M. Mendelsohn, M.D.

THE SYNTHESIS OF SELF

VOLUME 1
THE I OF CONSCIOUSNESS
Development from Birth to Maturity

ROY M. MENDELSOHN, M.D.

PLENUM MEDICAL BOOK COMPANY
NEW YORK AND LONDON

Library of Congress Cataloging in Publication Data

Mendelsohn, Roy M.
  The synthesis of self.

  Contents: v. 1. The I of consciousness—v. 2. It all depends on how you look at it—
v. 3. Believing is seeing—[etc.]
  Includes bibliographies and index.
  1. Self. 2. Psychology, Pathological. 3. Psychotherapy. I. Title. [DNLM: 1. Consciousness. 2. Personality Disorders. 3. Psychoanalytic Theory. 4. Psychoanalytic
Therapy—methods. WM 190 M537s]
RC455.4.S42M46 1987   616.89   87-25798

ISBN-13: 978-1-4612-9079-7   e-ISBN-13: 978-1-4613-1945-0
DOI: 10.1007/ 978-1-4613-1945-0

© 1987 Plenum Publishing Corporation
Softcover reprint of the hardcover 1st edition 1987
233 Spring Street, New York, N.Y. 10013

Plenum Medical Book Company is an imprint of Plenum Publishing Corporation

To my teachers:

my family who taught me to love,
Missy who taught me about autonomy,
Rebel who taught me about life,
and my patients who taught me what to write

Overview of *The Synthesis of Self*

This series consists of four volumes. Volume 1 addresses healthy development, moving from the earliest, most primitive stages to the most advanced stages, culminating in a picture of the genital character. The therapeutic progress of an autistic child is presented to illustrate the various developmental steps negotiated during the course of his treatment, supplemented by clinical material from others demonstrating similar points.

Volumes 2 and 3 address the pathological consequences of an inability to negotiate specific developmental tasks, moving from those with the most advanced psychic organization to those with the most primitive, culminating in a description of the autistic disorders. There was a natural division into two volumes owing to the crucial significance of cohesiveness for determining the conditions necessary to facilitate constructive growth. Some clinical material from Volume 1 is used to bring out the full picture of the pathology, which had only been alluded to in the earlier volume because of its focus on healthy processes.

Volume 4 addresses the basic principles of psychoanalytic treatment and their applicability across the broad spectrum of pathology, moving from the most primitive autistic disorders to the most advanced hysterical disturbances, to explicate the essence of the principles and their evolution into a classical psychoanalytic posture. Some clinical material from Volumes 1–3 is included to demonstrate the effects of the therapeutic relationship—when guided by the basic psychoanalytic principles in accordance with their essential nature—on both healthy and pathological processes.

The use of several patients' psychic productions throughout the series of four volumes illuminates the interweaving of healthy and pathological forces operative in a given individual, highlights their significance in guiding a therapist toward conducting a growth-promoting therapeutic relationship, and provides a thread of continuity connecting health, pathology, and treatment.

Roy M. Mendelsohn, M.D.
St. Louis

Preface

A psychoanalyst, through training and experience, directs the entire focus of his attention to registering and internalizing the input of a patient's communications, listening intently for their implied meanings. It is only by unraveling the mysteries of an unconscious realm of mental activity that it becomes possible to fully comprehend the way in which mental productions are finally observable. The psychoanalyst's total personality is the listening instrument, and the messages emanating from this hidden sector most clearly heard, deciphered, and understood are those most resonant with the contents of the psychoanalyst's unconscious. It is probable that a variety of psychoanalysts adopting a listening posture with a given patient would hear and understand a multiplicity of different meanings. Over the years, sensitive, well-trained psychoanalytic investigators have formulated concepts concerning mental functioning from disparate and often opposing points of view. These contradictory ideas are offered from a basic theoretical foundation placing unconscious mental events as the most important force shaping human experience. Divergent opinions may at times appear irreconcilable and then serve as the grounds for developing a separate psychoanalytic school of thought. It is not surprising that an exploration of unseen powerful and regressive forces, by a group of scientists with unique individual experiences, would yield insights sensitively attuned to a wide variety of important factors determining human development and behavior. It is this blend that challenges theoretical constructs, preventing them from becoming static, and furthers the expansion of knowledge.

The attitude required to gain enlightenment when entering dark areas of uncertainty in metapsychological theory is similar to what is needed in understanding the undiscovered reaches of a patient's internal world. The unfolding of new information cannot be obstructed by a need to impose unity, order, logic, or meaning, and there must be an ability to sift through and filter out the distortions created by pathology in order to elicit the kernels of truth that must flourish for growth to eventuate. Memory and desire operate as a hindrance to new learning and to the emergence of vulnerable unconscious truths that have been carefully defended against. A therapeutic attitude consistently embodies the implied question, How is the patient right? rather than making a determination of how the patient is wrong. In this way, underlying truths become more accessible to revelation, and their significance is more fully grasped. The theoretical formulations presented in this volume have been approached in a similar manner. The valuable contributions of instinctual theory, object relations theory, self psychological theory, and ego psychology are all taken into account, keeping the question of how they are right in the foreground.

A developmental perspective is given integrating these varied points of view, by outlining the mechanisms and processes involved in mental structure formation from birth to maturity, and defining the specific self- and object representations at the foundation of id, ego, and superego functions. Clinical examples illustrate each advancing step in psychic organization and constructive growth, highlighted by following the therapeutic progress of an autistic child. The interrelationship between perceptual processes and mental structure formation is formulated throughout with a detailed focus on the unfolding systems of consciousness and the perceptual agencies monitoring their regulatory principles. Libido is defined as object seeking rather than discharge seeking by identifying the original object of libidinal representation; this eliminates the concept of primary narcissism, which has been a source of confusion and extreme controversy. An exposition of the structural precursors of the superego is introduced, bringing clarity to the evolution and fate of the grandiose self and ego ideal. Fixation points are defined within a perceptual context that illuminates the means by which object constancy is maintained and character defenses are organized, creating the necessary preconditions for the emergence of an oedipal conflict. The organizing function of the oedipal situation is depicted, emphasizing its significance in negotiating the transition from narcissism to object relatedness. The important distinction between primal scene and incestuous fantasies is explained, and the alterations in the fixation points preparatory to replacing infantile attachments is discussed. A developmental line for the functioning of unconscious perceptions is elaborated, providing a sound theoretical basis for their guiding of the conduct of a therapeutic relationship.

Portions of Chapters 1 and 2 are reprinted from "The Onset of Unconscious Perception" by Roy M. Mendelsohn, 1985, *The Yearbook of Psychoanalysis and Psychotherapy*, Vol. 1, pp. 209–239. (Copyright 1985 by Lawrence Erlbaum Associates, Inc. Reprinted by permission.)

Roy M. Mendelsohn, M.D.

St. Louis

Contents

Contents of Other Volumes

Volume 2
It All Depends on How You Look at It:
Development of Pathology
in the Cohesive Disorders

Volume 3
Believing Is Seeing: Pathology of
Development in the Noncohesive Disorders

Volume 4
The Principles That Guide the Ideal Therapist

Introduction

It has always been recognized that to fully comprehend mental events it is essential to have a grasp of developmental lines and sequences. To do so requires an understanding of the earliest periods of mental development. This is a mental zone that can never be directly observed, and yet we know that it has a profound influence upon those mental productions that can be observed. We can make inferences from these more observable mental productions and attempt to validate our inferences in a variety of ways. However, these earliest realms of mental experience are almost totally latent. In addition, the manner in which these embryonic mental functions operate are in opposition to the modes of mental activities that are utilized in attempting to understand them. It is therefore important to be aware that the very effort to conceptualize and hypothesize about these earliest forms of mental functioning may create distortions in our manner of eliciting evidence of them and hence distort rather than clarify their essence.

The psychological contents of later developmental phases are more clearly observable, and grasping their significance may appear to be an easier task. The knowledge that they are based on a foundation that we understand little about complicates that task and emphasizes the importance of an ongoing exploration of these deeper, more primitive levels of experience. Any understanding of psychological experience that we attain is heavily dependent for validation upon the responses and reactions of the individual who has expressed them. The nature of what is considered to be validating varies according to the area of mental activity that we

1

are exploring. Manifest content is significant and reveals the functioning of the ego and the conscious to preconscious realms of mental activity. However, for a fuller understanding of a given event, it is essential to see its connection to latent content. In these later developmental phases, we gain that understanding once again from the individual who has expressed it but now with the added dimension of our subjective inferences. These are facilitated by the indirect or derivative expressions that illucidate the latent meaning. Latent content reveals the functioning of the unconscious system of mental activity. When we now attempt to hypothesize about the line of development of a given psychic event, it adds an even further dimension of complexity. This has been the most difficult area because, in the domain of the earliest phases of development, there is much uncertainty as to what is validating. A lot depends upon our subjective responses to the experiences we are participating in and observing. This puts special emphasis upon our individual ability to process subjective responses and to make use of our patients' mental productions in determining what is validating.

The proposals being offered in this presentation are based upon formulations covering these earliest phases of development. They are an attempt to conceptualize the developmental lines and sequences that evolve from the onset of human experience. The proposals being offered are therefore highly speculative and are abstractions and implications that have been drawn from experiences with patients. They seemed to have particular relevance for illuminating the connections of these earliest periods to later, more observable psychological phenomena.

Some years ago, when I was a beginning therapist, I saw a young boy who did nothing in his life or with me but sit, rock, and moan loudly. I saw him daily and spoke with him about many things, but his behavior never varied. At first, I put into words the theories I was learning as to the causes of his "illness." As time went on, these words felt empty and hollow to me, and my words slowly reflected my growing frustration and anguish. I spoke with a wise supervisor about my reactions and wondered how long I should keep working with the boy. The supervisor answered that I should continue as long as I felt the anguish and despair, and so I did. One day, after 8 months, this young boy spoke to me for the first time. I was startled as he told me of the little man on his shoulder shouting obscenities in his ears. That morning, the little man had spoken in a different voice, and so the boy could now talk. The little man's words were reflections of my words, especially the ones I uttered in my anguish and despair. In the years that followed, it was a revelation to me as this exquisitely sensitive child reacted to any defensive or pathological reaction on my part with the active return of this destructive man on his shoulder.

Since that time, I have had the opportunity of working with a small number of children who were regarded as being "autistic." These children clearly indicated their need for growth-producing experiences in the relationship with me. They sought out my weaknesses and vulnerability by attempting to engage me in pathological interactions, and whenever they succeeded, all communication ceased. They gradually taught me the characteristics that determined whether an interaction was healthy or pathological. As I learned, they became more articulate about themselves and more communicative about their inner and outer worlds. It then became possible for me to observe the manner in which their psychological growth proceeded. I was impressed at the degree to which my observations were consonant with, and evocative of, segments of articles and books I was reading. However, they also conflicted with other aspects of my reading, sometimes by the same author. It occurred to me that the processes and mechanisms of the earliest developmental phases were taking place right before my eyes.

When therapeutic contact was first initiated, it was extremely difficult to determine the composition of these children's mental representational worlds. Communication depended almost entirely upon my inferences, derived from their behavior. My subjective responses became a barometer of empathy, as they verbalized their internal experiences when I was sufficiently in tune to be trusted. It was then possible for me to note the degree to which mental representations had been fragmented, the vastness of the destructive impressions of an object, and the dearth of good self-experiences. These very primitive children slowly displayed a capacity to represent self-experience, to consolidate it into discrete entities determined by the presence or absence of defense, and to organize it into a system of self-representations. Concomitantly, the impressions of an object's influence were similarly represented, consolidated into entities, and organized into a functional system. In the context of the therapeutic relationship, mental structures were formed that united and differentiated the two systems of representation. One consequence was in the emergence of functional and adaptive capacities that were also displayed in their attitudes and interactions with other people and in other situations. I was able to observe how differing aspects of self-experience and of an object's influence coalesced from part self- and part object representations into a whole unit. Many authors had written about the consolidation of part self- and part object representations into a whole self and whole object. The experience I was having seemed to shed some light upon this process that I had not seen described in an integrated and consistent fashion. Initially, I did not know whether my observations were a product of the unique development of these children or whether what transpired was a consequence of their original pathology. After having similar experiences with other children, I began to wonder if I might be seeing processes that were following a sequence of steps that reflected the earliest periods in human psychological development. I also found that my understanding of others was enhanced and broadened by what I was discovering with this group of children. They made me aware of how vital it is for any therapeutic endeavor to be based upon a relatively solid foundation of healthy interactional qualities that are sensitively attuned to what is needed by a given patient. In this presentation, I have focused upon the characteristics of healthy development from birth to maturity. I have only referred to pathological outcomes when it served to more clearly outline the functioning of healthy processes.

I have spent some time considering the significance of these experiences and synthesizing them with my readings in the literature. I paid particular attention to the writings that influenced my thinking and noted some similarities and differences with what those authors had hypothesized.

Jacobson (1964), in her important work, *The Self and the Object World*, provided a conceptual framework for a deeper understanding of early development. Along with Hartman (1939) and others, she went far in defining the differences between ego, self, and self-representations. I have defined the self exclusively from a perceptual point of view and delineated the role of perception in activating the representational and organizational functions of the ego. Varied aspects of perceptual experience are consolidated and organized into discrete entities that create two functional systems of mental representation. One is composed of body ego experiences that are represented to form a system of self-representations. The other is composed of their object-impression counterparts that are represented to form a system of object representations. These mental events take place within boundaries, established by the activity of perception, that determine the concept of a self. The sequence of developmental steps that must be negotiated for the tripartite structures of id, ego, and superego to ultimately form and operate within these boundaries will be described.

Many authors, beginning with Freud (1938/1964), have emphasized the importance of a body ego experience as the foundation for every mental event. This concept has been generally well accepted. However, there has been some difficulty in appreciating its significance. For example, the experience of identity and of autonomy are later developments that are observable. This implies that, at the outset of development, there exists a core body ego experience of separateness that is at the foundation of the sense of autonomy and identity. The primitively organized children, to whom I referred earlier, all initially displayed a body ego experience of objectlessness. In the course of their progression to more advanced levels of psychic organization, this core of objectlessness evolved into an inner sense of identity and autonomy. A lack of differentiation was manifested but only during the time when mental representations of self-experience and of an object's influence elicited by the therapeutic relationship were forming. The lack of differentiation was an intermediary step from objectlessness to autonomy and appeared to be essential for the processes of introjection and internalization to occur. This developmental sequence and the subsequent self-expansion were immediately evocative of Mahler's (1958) descriptions of a psychological symbiosis. It underscores the need to conceptualize the specific body ego experiences that underlie the observable functions of later developmental periods.

Jacobson's work was affected by the limitations in ego psychological theory available to her at the time. She displayed a tendency to make giant leaps in formulating the sequential steps of developmental processes. In addition, there was an insufficient definition of the mechanisms involved in each step that was described. Jacobson (1964) referred to the formation of self- and object representations, but her descriptions of the alternating fluctuation of processes of fusion and differentiation were overgeneralized and vague. However, her formulations went far toward integrating object relations theory into the main body of instinctual theory and into a psychology of the ego. My patients indicated that body ego experiences and their object-impression counterparts possessed sufficiently different qualities so that they were represented separately. Furthermore, these part self- and part object representations coalesced to form consolidated entities in accordance with the need for, or presence of, defense. Self-experiences that did not require defense were represented as facets of a whole good self and consisted of (1) phase-specific instinctual gratifications, (2) the body ego experiences evoked by utilizing autonomous ego functions, and (3) the body ego experience resulting from perceptual contact with the intrauterine environment. This latter aspect has been beautifully protrayed by Grotstein (1981) and called "the background object of primary identification." Self-experiences that required or included defense were represented as facets of a whole bad self and consisted of (1) instinctual overstimulation, (2) body ego experiences of sensory deprivation, and (3) the reactions to impingements.

Object relations theorists have advanced our understanding of the significance of interactions with the external world. The effects of these interactions upon the intrapsychic processes of structuralization, during the early phases of development, have been a matter of controversy. The insights gained have had fragmentary value and have suffered from an inability to develop a metapsychology that incorporates object relations theory with instinctual theory, ego psychological theory, and a theory of the psychology of the self. Some of the difficulty has been created from the concept of libido as discharge seeking, rather than as object seeking. Libidinal theory was formulated prior to structural theory and was never fully revised. In recent years it has become evident that revision is necessary. The idea of libido as discharge seeking can be maintained in explaining the complex functions that are observed in the later phases of psychosexual development. When an attempt is made to trace the developmental line of a given, more advanced mental structure, it becomes apparent that libido is involved with an object at each step. Kohut (1971) attempted to deal with this observation by postulating two separate lines of narcissistic development. In any exploration of the intrapsychic events and interactional processes that further self-expansion, it is essential to include formulations as to the mechanisms involved in interactions with the external world and the manner in which they are represented in the internal world. Fairbairn (1954), in response to this difficulty, had to develop a theory of object relations that eliminated instinctual theory. His rationale evolved from the observation that libido appeared to be object seeking from the outset of development. This was a serious deficiency because libidinal theory has shed so much light upon the psychosexual experiences of human beings throughout the course of their lives.

Another area of confusion and controversy has centered around the development of the superego. Some of the difficulty is in the lack of a clear delineation of the precursors of superego formation. A need exists to trace the developmental line and identify the original body ego experience, operating as a foundation, for the organization of the superego as a functional psychic agency relatively independent of interactions with the external world. Jacobson (1964) and others have presented a definition of the differences between the genetic precursors in the development of the superego and the emergence of the superego as an independently functioning psychic structure. However, the sequential steps in this development were not clearly elaborated. In addition, there has been confusion and lack of clarity in discussions of wishful self- and object images and realistic self- and object images. Hartmann (1962) noted the early emergence of magical, idealizing, wishful fantasies that ultimately consolidated into the ego ideal aspect of the superego. The processes, mechanisms, motivations, and sequential steps of this evolution were left open for speculation. Jacobson (1964) similarly leaves this facet of development unclarified. Although she describes the transformation of wishful self- and object images into real self- and object images, she does not describe the manner by which this significant change takes place.

The adaptive point of view, elaborated by Hartmann (1939), was vital for constructing a developmental psychology of the ego. This exposition opened the doors to exploring the interrelationship of developing ego functions and the adaptive task of interacting with the external environment. The manner in which the ego and its functions adapt to the demands of the internal and external worlds have a profound effect upon the functions themselves and upon the mental structures that are formed as a result of their functioning. Hartmann's theoretical formulations gave impetus to the task of tracing the developmental lines of specific ego functions, the processes that enhance or interfere with them, and the influences of interactions with the external world. A deeper perspective on the role of energic differentiation also became possible. These theoretical ideas were of inestimable value in attaining an ever-broadening view of the psychology of the ego. Others, particularly Jacobson (1964), attempted to fill in gaps in the understanding of early development by specifying the self- and object representational structures that participated in the maturation of ego functions.

Throughout the literature, there has been a lack of clarification as to the significance, the evolution, the fate, or even the existence of the structure of the grandiose self. In particular, there have been only fragmentary references to the important developmental function that this structure provides. Often, the grandiose self is not identified as a developmentally significant structure. When it is, there is no elucidation of a relationship to other facets of development or of its fate as the ego ideal gains in predominance. The concept of a grandiose self has been an evocative focus for theory formation. The universal presence of wishful self- and object imagery in human experience has been a stimulus for efforts to conceptualize its lines of development. There has been uncertainty expressed as the whether it is a healthy or pathological structure or in regard to its ultimate fate throughout the life cycle. The discussions, though infused with controversy, have called attention to the concept of the grandiose self as having the potential for a synthesis of the findings of the ego psychologists with the observations of the object relations theorists. Some authors, Kohut (1971), for example, consider the formation of the grandiose self as a basic developmental step. In Kohut's conception of the formation of a bipolar self, the grandiose self emerges as an expression of one pole of the self. Kernberg (1980) conceptualizes the grandiose self as an intrapsychic structure that functions to organize specific pathological states. The manner in which wishful imagery is transformed into realistic imagery has been either inadequately explained, contradictory explanations are given, or it is described with the implication that it is self-evident. In the writings of Kohut (1971) and Kernberg (1980), these wishful images are defined as a manifestation of the grandiose self. However, there are confused and contradictory expositions concerning its formation. The relationship of the grandiose self to earlier developmental processes and its fate in later periods are never clearly formulated. There is uncertainty as to how, or even whether, it is modified to meet the demands of reality testing. There is also no reference to the fate of the grandiose self when its influence is no longer openly evident. I have viewed the grandiose self as a mental structure that is formed to unite and differentiate the self- and object systems of representation at a specific point in development. That point is reached when the experiences of helplessness and vulnerability, associated with the recognition of separateness, motivates the need for an object's influence that will provide balance. The structured union is based upon participation in a fantasy of the object's omnipotence, and hence I have called it "the grandiose self." I will discuss the evolution, effect, function, and fate of the grandiose self throughout the life cycle. I will also discuss the relationship of the grandiose self to the formation of another structure—the ego ideal. This is a structure founded upon the process of selective identification, in which admired qualities of an object are included within self-experience. The interrelationship of these two structures solidifies the cohesiveness of self-experience and explicates the means by which wishful imagery is transformed into realistic imagery. The interdependent relationship between perceptual functions and mental representation is depicted throughout the body of this work and is elaborated upon to demonstrate how perceptual boundaries are established within the personality. The perceptual functions incorporated in the structuralization of the grandiose self and ego ideal play an integral part in the organization of the superego as an independent agency. I will attempt to provide clarification by depicting the lines and sequences of development that eventuate in the formation of the grandiose self, explore the relationship of the grandiose self and ego ideal, and describe the fate of these structures throughout the life cycle.

Jacobson (1964) hypothesized a short-lasting state of primary narcissism at the outset of development, prior to the formation of a representational world. She referred to it as a psychophysiological state of the self. The initial representation of the self and object are poorly differentiated and are reflective of a symbiotic interaction. Jacobson pointed out that once a representation has formed, the state of primary narcissism no longer exists. Implicit in this formulation is that the lack of differentiation between representations of the self and object is a developmental advance. It also implies that there is an underlying body ego experience, present at birth, of contact with an object that is simultaneously inside and outside of the self. Jacobson felt the concept of primary masochism was unnecessary because the original undifferentiated energy state is only identified as libidinal or aggressive when structures are available to represent it. She continued to postulate an original state of primary narcissism but indicated that it was so short lasting as to be insignificant as a concept. In my opinion, the concept of primary narcissism is not only unnecessary for an understanding of psychic events but is inaccurate and confusing. There is much evidence to indicate that perceptual processes function *in utero*, which would be the basis for a primitive interaction with the intrauterine environment. This intrauterine experience is the foundation for representing what Grotstein (1981) has called "the background object of primary identification." It is the body ego experience of contact with an object that establishes the necessary background for a psychological symbiosis. Kernberg (1980), Jacobson (1964), Mahler (1958), and others have hypothesized an initial phase in which self and objects can not yet be differentiated. Object relations theorists, particularly Klein (1955), Fairbairn (1954), and Bion (1968), have indicated that, at the outset, there is a phase of primitive objectless differentiation. It requires developmental progression, through the effects of an empathic interaction with an external object, for a lack of differentiation to evolve. This lack of differentiation fosters the experiences of fusion and merger that are essential for representations of the self and object to be elaborated. This concept underscores Freud's (1938/1964) description of the original ego as a body ego under the dominance of a reality principle. It is only with advances in development and the formation of self- and object representations that the pleasure principle can begin to assert itself. Later, with sufficient structuralization, there is a return to the dominance of the reality principle in a new way.

Jacobson (1964) utilized the concept of object relationships in a specific fashion. The formation of self-and object representations are presented as stages in development that must be negotiated to establish an object relationship. Jacobson regarded an object relationship as a complex task of recognition. It referred to the perception of an object in the outside world, separate from the self, and having objects of its own. This means that the ability to form an object relationship depends upon the intrapsychic capacity to achieve that perception. The earlier stages reflect a narcissistic orientation to stimuli, which has a very different effect upon the way in which external interactions are represented. I believe this distinction is important, for clarity, in discerning the influence of external objects. The particular manner in which a stimulus is registered and the meaning it is given are determined by the level of psychic organization that has been attained. In the course of healthy development, a shift takes place, from a narcissistic to an object-related perspective, which is manifested in the ability to perceive the object as having independent objects of its own. This change in perspective is an integral part of the elaboration of an oedipal conflict, which creates the structural foundation for object-related perceptions to be realized. It is thus important to conceptualize the original body ego experience that operate as a background for that perceptual capacity to emerge.

I have developed a concept that calls attention to the significance of biophysiological demands and the effects of bodily processes as an ongoing source of stimulation within the organism. Although biophysiological demands are present on a continuum, they are registered by the perceptual processes and represented in accordance with their degree of intensity. The dimension that does not require defense is represented as an aspect of good self-experience, and as intensity mounts and defenses are activated, it is represented as an aspect of bad self-experience. Another dimesion has the perceptual impact of an impingement, cannot be contained within the self-experience, and leaves the impression of an overstimulating instinctual object. Finally, there is a dimension on the continuum that is unperceivable and cannot be represented. I have called this continuum of biophysiologic demand "the self with object qualities" because it is a part of the self and possesses the independent qualities of an object. A number of authors have called attention to the almost universal existence of a level of regressive functioning that, under certain conditions, can reach psychotic proportions. This phenomenon has been described by Balint (1968) as "the basic fault" and by Bion (1968) as "the psychotic sector of the personality." Although it is a common clinical observation, there has not been a clear exposition as to its place in the sequential scheme of development. I will portray the significance of the dimension on the continuum of instinctual demand that is present as a force within the organism but is incapable of representation and remains outside of the self. The impact of this stimulus upon the primitive psyche, its effect upon succeeding phases of development, and the sequential steps of psychic structuralization that have to be negotiated for it to be included and integrated within self-experience will be explicated. It is not until the capacity to perceive an object as having unseen objects of its own has developed that this aspect can attain access to representation. If this traumatic intensity of biophysiological demand is too vigorously defended against initially, it may remain inaccessible to the integrative pathways that are structured as personality organization progresses. The ability to represent increasing amounts of biophysiologic demand in reflected in the advancing stages of development of the component instincts. Within this narcissistic organization, the unseen dimension is traumatic and cannot be represented. This is the area of the personality described by Balint (1968) as "the basic fault" and by Bion (1968) as "the psychotic sector." The consolidation of the component instincts into a genital drive is associated with an intensification of instinctual activity that motivates the organization of a new level of psychic structuralization. Perceptual contact with the self with object qualities establishes the original body ego experience that is necessary as a foundation to register the perception of external objects. The oedipal conflict organizes new structures that enable the representation of the unseen dimension on the continuum of biophysiological demand. This serves as a foundation for the perception that an external object has unseen objects of its own.

A major fault in Jacobson's (1964) *The Self and the Object World* is the confusion in her use of the concepts of *repression proper, primal repression,* and the early infantile defenses of *denial* and *splitting.* Kernberg (1980) defined the self, object, and affect unions that comprise mental structures and delineated the mechanism of splitting in early development. He emphasized the pathological consequences when this mechanism operates beyond its phase-appropriate stages. However, his descriptions tended to be static and mechanical and did not portray the means by which splitting mechanisms were healed. I will utilize a perceptual point of view to explain the significance of splits within the ego, describe the conditions and motives that determine their ascendency as a primary defense, and trace their fate in later phases of development. *Splitting* will be defined as a translocation of perception, in which a given stimulus is represented away from its source. I will explicate the reasons for this perceptual translocation and the means by which stimuli can be represented at their source, as the splits are healed.

Psychoanalytic authors have attempted to be discerning in the determination of how an external object's influence can be instrumental in the growth and expansion of the representational world. Jacobson (1964), for example, defined the concepts of introjection, primitive identification, and selective identification in an effort to discriminate between intrapsychic mechanisms operating at differing levels of psychic organizations. In her definition, *primitive identifications* referred to the poorly differentiated fusions of self- and object images. In later phases of development, when the representations of self and object are differentiated, aspects of the object are incorporated within the representations of the self. Jacobson described this process as one of introjection and used it interchangeably with selective identification. Her tendency to focus exclusively upon intrapsychic events and her use of *introjection* and *selective identification* as synonymous terms seemed to make it difficult to make use of the insights of object relations theory. In my view, *introjection* refers to the process of registering a stimulus and is at the foundation of all perceptual experiences from the most primitive to the most advanced. *Primitive identifications* would encompass the fusion of self- and object images within a symbiosis but would need to specify the aspects of self-experience that are expanded by empathic resonance with an external object. *Selec-*

tive identifications require the presence of a well-differentiated system of object representations and involve the process of including admired qualities of an object within the self-experience. A full understanding of any mental activity requires an explication of the original body ego experience that serves as an underlying foundation, and after which it is modeled. This is especially difficult in regard to the process of internalization, which is initiated with the dawning of existence. However, a theoretical grasp of these earliest stages in development is essential to establish a line of continuity with later, more demonstrable phenomena. It is thus important to formulate a theoretical construct illucidating an embryonic experience of contact with an object that is simultaneously inside and outside of the self.

I have engaged in such a venture, by postulating the emergence of a nuclear self with the awakening of perceptual functions *in utero*. In this primordial state, stimuli are registered at two locales. One is at the interior, the point of perceptual contact with the demands of biophysiology; the second is at the periphery, the point of perceptual contact with the intrauterine environment. At both sites, a primitive body ego experience is represented, in which the stimulus is at one and the same time both inside and outside of the nuclear self. The continuum of biophysiological demand has a dimension that is outside of the primitively organized boundaries of the self, yet inside of the organism. The metabolizing, containing, physiologic functions of the intrauterine surround are registered as simultaneously inside and outside of the nuclear self and are represented as the background object of primary identification. The latter serves as a model for all subsequent processes of identification and establishes the background for engaging in the psychological symbiosis of postuterine life. It is a representation of self-experience that does not require defense; it is formed as the result of contact with an object; and it is available as the initial object for the representation of instinctual activity. This conceptual framework allows libido to be formulated as object seeking and eliminates the idea of an early phase of primary narcissism.

Jacobson (1964) postulated an original undifferentiated state of instinctual energy. She deemed the concept of primary masochism and a death instinct as no longer essential to explain the various phenomena related to the aggressive drives. She also believed the concept of primary narcissism was of limited usefulness. She pointed out that the self-representations are treated by the instincts as an object. Because there must be engagement with an object for a self-representation to form and because instincts are in an undifferentiated state until there is a mental representation available to identify them as libidinal or aggressive, narcissism is secondary. Jacobson added that the concept of primary narcissism could still be applicable to the limited time prior to the establishment of a self-representation. The concept of libido as discharge seeking has stood as a major obstacle in the pathway of integrating the contributions of object relations theory into the main body of psychoanalytic metapsychology. It is also vital for grounding the clinical observation that progress in psychoanalytic treatment is most strongly influenced by the nature of the interaction. In the body of this presentation, as I outline the advancing stages of psychosexual development, I will be synthesizing object relations theory, instinctual theory, and a psychology of the self from a perceptual (ego psychological) point of view.

The concept of *primary narcissism* was responsible for Kohut's (1971) hypothesis of a separate line of narcissistic development. He postulated the existence of a "bipolar self." At one pole, ambitions and goals emerge in response to the mirroring activities of an empathic external object. At the other pole, the self is narcissistically enhanced by the idealization of an object that leads to the emergence of morals and standards. Kohut defined healthy narcissism as the utilization of the individual's unique talents and skills, motivated by ambitions and goals, and regulated by morals and standards. He formulated these ideas from his experience in the psychoanalytic treatment of a particular group of patients that he diagnosed as having a narcissistic personality disorder. The patients he described exhibited these narcissistic qualities in their transference reactions. Kohut felt that it was vital for these narcissistic transferences to flourish and that the empathic responsiveness of the analyst would foster their emergence in the treatment situation. The analyst's empathy would be conveyed through interpretations of the patients' developmental need. Interpretations, of reactions to inevitable lapses in empathy, would result in a process of transmuting internalization. In this way, new structures could form, and the arrested lines of narcissistic development could progress within the transference relationship. The therapist's task would be to provide mirroring to the self if the defect were at that pole of the self, or to facilitate the process of idealization if the compensatory activities at that pole of the self needed to be enhanced. Healing would take place by the repair of narcissistic defects and result in a cohesive self. I will formulate a sequence of development that places the clinical observations Kohut made reference to in a different perspective. It will define the self on a different basis and obviate the idea of a separate line of narcissistic development.

The different explanation is based upon the idea that libido is object seeking and that primary narcissism is a nonuseful concept. The process of engagement with an object begins *in utero* and establishes a body ego experience, represented as the background object of primary identification, which is the foundation for the psychological symbiosis in postuterine life. This part self-representation serves as the first object of libidinal activity in the earliest stages of development. I will detail the formation of two functional systems of representations, which could be described as a bipolar self. At one pole, body ego experiences coalesce into a system of self-representations. At the other pole, their object-impression counterparts coalesce into a system of object representations. Ambitions and goals are based upon self-experiences, morals and standards are based upon the influences of an object, and the utilization of talents and skills depends upon a harmonious interrelationship between the two realms of experience. Thus the description by Kohut of healthy narcissism can be more effectively understood as the manifestation of a healthy, functional superego operating in harmony with the interests of the ego. I will discuss the sequences, mechanisms, and processes by which self-cohesiveness and self-expansion take place. The implications for what constitutes empathy in the therapist will also be addressed. There is a significant difference between an empathic response to conscious and unconscious experience because unconscious perceptions and fantasies can only be expressed through derivatives. An explication of the process by which derivatives are formed and of their representational foundation is essential as a background for unconscious empathy.

Some authors have conceived of the ego as embedded within the self; others have presented the self as embedded in the ego. This presentation emphasizes the role of perception in determining self-experience and in forming the boundaries within which it is represented. Perceptual processes activate the representational and organizational functions of the ego, which ultimately eventuates in the consolidation and unification of two discrete, well-differentiated functional systems of mental representations. One, the self-system, is based upon body ego experiences. The other, the object system, is based upon their object-impression counterparts. An interdependent relationship is established between perception and the functional systems of representation to attain progressively advanced levels of psychic organization. I will describe the sequential steps involved in defining the circumscribed structural entities of id, ego, and superego and the manner in which the varied systems of consciousness are delineated. The self then emerges as a supraordinate concept.

The title of this work, *The I of Consciousness*, stresses the significance of the self (I) and of experience (consciousness). The title is also meant to allude to "the eye of consciousness." Mental events, which are multidetermined and exposed to numerous influences, reveal the forces that have shaped them through the manner in which they are perceived. Hoffer (1952) and Spitz (1955) stressed the idea that the perceptual processes function as psychic organizers. These authors constructed a theoretical framework for tracing the effects of early developmental processes upon later mental productions. Both authors focused on the role of perception, but their speculations appear to be contradictory. This may be partly due to the adultomorphic effect of any attempt to describe the early events of infantile life. The contradictory ideas concern the high priority given to the representation of visual experience during the earliest stages of forming a representational world. The optic tracts are the last to attain myelinization, and in the maturational sequence of perceptual modalities, visual processes are the last to register their activities on the representational functions of the ego. The near receptors of touch, smell, and taste, which are closer to body ego experience, have a greater impact on the ego's representational functions and exert their activities earlier. The distance receptors of hearing and sight have a greater impact on the ego's organizational functions and exert their activities at a later time. Consensual validation is established when the various perceptual modalities are integrated as a functional unit. This means that the ability of the near receptors to evoke representational functions is available to the distance receptors and that the ability of the distance receptors to evoke organizational functions is available to the near receptors. The consolidation of part self-experiences into whole entities occurs concomitantly with the integration of perceptual functions and coincides temporally with the capacity to perceive the self and object as separate. The interrelationship of perceptual activity and mental structure formation is reflected in the function of self-observation. It is based upon the structured representation of the internal search for a separate good object's influence—the eye of consciousness. This focused area of perceptual activity registers mental events in a visual modality and is indicative of the establishment of consensual validation.

Bion (1968) described the early processes of introjection and projective identification. He presented a vivid portrayal of the fantasies involved in these processes and of their effect on the course of continuing development. He depicted the infant's capacity to fantasy the projections of parts of the self into the object, and conversely, to incorporate parts of the object into the self. However, he did not delineate the underlying representations of self-experience and of an object's influence that are necessary as a base for fantasies to develop. He also did not explain the motive for their formation or the means by which fantasies become available to engage in processes of introjection and projective identification. I will attempt to fill in this gap by demonstrating that each body ego experience and each impression of an object is elaborated into specific fantasies and that each fantasy serves a particular purpose that is determined by its composition. This provides a basis for illuminating the interplay of internal and external forces that are shaping the personality and for identifying the motives and pathways of introjective and projective mechanisms. Fantasy elaborations are formulated as mental productions whose function is to link the self- and object systems of representations. Bion (1968) introduced the idea of the destruction of linkages as being a primary force in the production of pathology, by virtue of the resulting destruction of meaning. This important concept did not offer a definition of meaning that could shed light upon specifically what was destroyed and upon the processes involved in its destruction. A definition of the creation of meaning would clarify the manner in which it evolves and is destroyed. It is my impression that three component parts must be present for meaning to occur. These are a representation of self-experience, a representation of an object's influence, and a fantasy that links one to the other. The manner in which meaning is developed, interfered with, distorted, or destroyed is then dependent upon the internal and external conditions that enhance or interfere with the formation of this union. The specific qualities in an interaction that foster the destruction of meaning, obviate against its destruction, or enhance its evolution become more evident. Kernberg (1980) defined the basic units of mental structure, as unions of self, object, and affect, which is consonant with this definition of meaning. However, he did not describe the developmental lines of each component.

Winnicott's (1958) characterization of the transitional object has had ever-broadening implications. The significance of a transitional object reaches far beyond its surface description as an object in the external world, having qualities of its own that can be shaped to serve a bridge between the self and the influences of a good object. In having the effect of evoking memory traces of a good object, it points to the presence of an original nidus around which varied impressions of a good object have coalesced. It tends to corroborate the idea of a primitive nuclear self forming *in utero*, in which the object-impression counterpart of the background object of primary identification is ultimately represented as a transitional object. A theoretical explanation will be presented as to its importance in establishing the foundation for a system of object representations and of the role of its fantasy elaborations in forming transitional space.

There has been much written about the similarities and differences between male and female development. I will approach this topic by describing the differences in the body ego experiences of males and females, the resulting effects upon self- and object representational structures, and the manner in which the oedipal situation and its resolution are shaped. I will include the role of gender identity within the total fabric of the processes of identification and identity formation. Jacobson (1964) called attention to earlier descriptions of women's having defective superegos, which were based upon women's fantasies of the absence of a phallus as a castration or defect. She referred to the woman's superego as different, not defective, and hypothesized the ego ideal forming at an earlier stage. In her view, it required a longer period of time for the wishful aspects of the ego ideal to be transformed into a more realistic self-image. I will attempt to clarify the different structural composition of the grandiose self and ego ideal and the nature of their interrelationship. Jacobson's portrayal of the early ego ideal is more aptly seen as an expression of the grandiose self. The idea of the grandiose self's operating as a dominant force for a longer time, within the developing feminine personality, is consistent with the female's greater capacity to integrate instinctual demands and greater difficulty in establishing feminine identifications. The female's phallically determined experience of disappointment in the mother, in conjunction with the evolving feeling of rivalry, makes the process of identification more difficult. Fantasies, in women, of the genitals being defective or damaged are certainly abundantly evident. However, they are based upon representations of self-experience and an object's influence that must be defined to determine their significance. I will discuss the differing manifestations of castration anxiety in males and females, which reflect the differences in the body ego experiences of genital excitation. The male shows greater difficulty in integrating instinctual demands and greater facility in establishing masculine identifications. I will define the negative oedipal constellation as a developmental step in the female and as a reflection of pathology in the male. This formulation differs from what some authors, such as Blos (1979), have written.

A background of knowledge concerning early development is essential for understanding the period of pubescence. Blos (1979) has called it ''a period of regression in the service of development.'' This has reference to the observation that earlier developmental steps are repeated at this later time. The accessibility of integrative functions, associated with a more advanced level of psychic organization, can be brought to achieving a resolution of earlier difficulties. It is during pubescence when primary infantile attachments to an object are replaced with the representations of independent attachments to new objects. Although this occurrence has been documented often, the specific means by which it takes place and the sectors of the personality that are involved are confusing and controversial. I have attempted to shed light upon the negotiation of this developmental task and to indicate the fate of the infantile representations that are replaced.

In the early history of psychoanalysis, emphasis was placed on the discovery of unconscious mental processes. The early literature was replete with illucidations of the psychology of the id. In the excitement of discovery, there was a tendency to either ignore or to not fully appreciate the significance of the developing ego. This was particularly true in regard to the effects of external interactions upon intrapsychic experience and upon the formation of mental representations. Later, attention was turned to an understanding of the psychology of the ego and of the developmental sequences of the various ego functions. A deeper grasp of the influence of external interactions emerged. It took a long period of time to appreciate the profound impact that interactional processes had upon human experience. In recent years, there has been a clearer delineation of the role that introjective and projective processes play in early structure formation. The expanded understanding of the mechanism of projective identification has broadened our awareness of the effects of the therapeutic interaction. Analysts have always known of the importance of countertransference responses but have disagreed as to the exact nature of their effects. There has been a tendency to attribute a patient's perceptions of a therapist almost solely to transference distortions. Concomitantly, the tendency is to not fully appreciate the validity and significance of a patient's unconscious perceptions. The confusion in this area, in part, is a result of the absence of a theoretical substrate on which to base a distinction between transference distortions (based on fantasy) and unconscious perceptions (based on body ego experience). In practice, every therapist knows of the significance of a patient's unconscious perceptions, although they might not be identified as such because the verification of interpretive interventions depends upon the derivative reactions and responses.

Earlier, I referred to the impetus for my writing. It was stimulated by my therapeutic experiences with a number of children described as autistic. These were children who were viewed as divorced from the external world of reality and as having shut out all human relationships. I began my therapeutic work with them, and it appeared quite different. They taught me, in some painful ways, that at times I unwittingly offered them a pathological relationship. On each occasion that I did so, they did in fact close me out. It was specifically at these moments that they were divorced from a human relationship. When I displayed any willingness or capacity to examine the part I played in the interaction, they would begin to communicate with me. At the time, this was a startling revelation that had a profound effect. It confronted me with the task of exploring my own motivations whenever these children ceased communication. Each time that I did, I was immensely rewarded with human communication from children who otherwise would not communicate at all. It alerted me to the realization that I had been explaining the differences in these children and other patients, as the difference between individuals who were analyzable and those who possessed what I thought of as ego deficits or developmental arrests. I gradually became aware of the powerful influence pathological or defensive responses on my part were having on the therapeutic process with all of my patients. With the children I described, the effect was immediate, concrete, and impossible to deny. With others, it was more subtle, elusive, and easy to rationalize.

For the past 10 years, Langs (1977) has been writing voluminously about the significance of the therapeutic interaction. He has stressed the idea that the management of the framework and ground rules of psychotherapy reflect the therapist's healthy and pathological functioning. He has emphasized the role of patients' encoded derivatives and unconscious perceptions. He has developed an intellectual framework for establishing a listening process that can distinguish between expressions of transference distortions and of unconscious perceptions. The unconscious perceptions of a patient can then be a guide and supervisor for the therapist. His work, however, has not been well grounded in developmental theory. The concepts offered in the body of this presentation provide the missing theoretical basis for Langs's observations. A developmental approach is adopted to explicate the foundation of unconscious perceptions and the evolution of varied systems of consciousness. A developmental line for the formation of derivatives is given definition, which aids in distinguishing between those expressing the effects of unconscious fantasies and those expressing the effects of unconscious perceptions. The qualities in an interaction that foster growth emerge within a developmental context and add clarity to the particular ingredients that constitute a constructive influence.

I will begin with a description and definition of the nuclear self. Particular emphasis will be placed on the role of perception in activating the representational and organizational functions of the ego to initiate the process of psychic structuralization. The importance of body ego experiences, and their object-impression counterparts, for consolidating self- and object systems of representation, is outlined. The concepts of "the self with object qualities" and "the object with self-qualities" are stressed throughout the body of this work, in conjunction with an exposition of the reciprocal relationship that is established between perception and mental representation. Splitting, as an early mechanism available to the ego, is given a perceptual definition. Its initial function in furthering differentiation and defense is detailed, as are the means by which these early splits in the ego heal. The motives that lead up to the formation of the grandiose self and ego ideal, which structuralize a differentiated union between the two systems of representation, are delineated. I have given a detailed description of the evolution, composition, function, and fate of these structures. The significance and makeup of fixation points is portrayed, as is their role in self-expansion. I have offered a theoretical basis for considering libido as object seeking, and in this context I have described the development of the component instincts and their consolidation into a genital drive. The emergence of castration anxiety as a signaling and regulatory structure, preparatory to the elaboration of an oedipal conflict, is illucidated. The manner in which the oedipal conflict serves as a psychic organizer is a significant aspect of this study and is coordinated with the consolidation of the superego into an independently functioning agency. Attention is directed throughout to the sequence of developmental events and its importance in understanding the hierarchical organization of the id of the dynamic unconscious. Changes in the fixation points that occur during the latency period are discussed, as is the crucial task of maintaining a structured pathway for the integration of instinctual demand. The events of pubescence are explicated, which includes an explanation of the similarities and differences in male and female development, with particular attention paid to the process of replacing the infantile attachments to primary objects. Each step in development is dependent upon the preceding steps, and the manner in which earlier steps influence a progressive step is explained. The qualities that comprise a genital character and their manifestations in work, play, and love mark the completion of this volume.

I have tended to write in a circular fashion, as I moved forward to a succeeding phase of development. With each repetition, I have attempted to broaden the significance of an idea by approaching it from a different perspective or by adding another dimension of meaning. I hope what is sacrificed in redundancy is made up for in depth of understanding. The essence of this work has been to synthesize instinctual theory, object relations theory, and a psychology of the self from an ego psychological (perceptual) point of view.

CHAPTER 1

Body Ego Experience and the Nuclear Self

The Onset of Unconscious Perception

Introduction

The expression that "seeing is believing" reflects a commonly held view that it is only that which is seen in concrete form that is believable. The expression could be reversed and have equal validity. The expression would become, "you have to believe in order to see." This reflects upon the myriad of experiences that pass unnoticed and depend for their observation on the particular belief of the observer. The earliest phases of developmental experience are unseeable in the usual sense and depend greatly upon the belief of the observer to be identified. A developmental line that can be traced to the onset of perceptual experience is necessary in order to fully comprehend the profound influence that people have upon each other. In this way, our view of what is healthy and constructive in human interactions can be broadened and expanded. One crucial dimension of my experience has centered around the realization that many of my patients were consciously unable to sort out the genuine responses that were growth producing from those that were unreal and destructive. Unconsciously, these same patients were exquisitely sensitive to these qualities. It seemed to me that many had become ill from the influence of the poisonous interactions operating in concert with, and dominating, healthy ones. It also seemed to me that my primary task was to slowly understand what had occurred and to learn through our therapeutic interaction to sort out the two, so that the patient's growth could continue. It appears to me that every human experience has the potential for being linked through its developmental line to the onset of its formation. In this chapter, I would like to address the processes, mechanisms, and the sequences of the earliest phases of structure formation at the foundation of unconscious perceptions. I will begin by presenting a concept of the nuclear self that is defined by the activity of perceptual processes and enlarge upon its significance. The original body ego experiences, by which a stimulus outside of the self is included through representation within the self, will be explicated to give a developmental foundation for the role of unconscious perceptions in an interaction. The effects of the therapist's interpretive activities, when they are based upon empathic responses to unconscious communications and when they are based upon empathic failures, will be explored. These effects are illustrative of the manner in which unconscious perceptions are manifested in a therapeutic interaction.

Clinical Material

A was a wizened-looking, 4-year-old boy with no identifiable communicative speech and only occasional singsong vocalizations. He wandered unendingly from place to place and submissively complied to external physical directions. He was referred, after being diagnosed on several occasions, as autistic, brain damaged, and/or retarded. He was seen in a series of diagnostic sessions to determine whether psychotherapeutic intervention was feasible and/or to aid the family in decision making concerning his future. The family had been advised that institutionalization was necessary, and the only question was when. In the first two sessions occurring on consecutive days, A stood silently and then awkwardly moved from place to place, gesturing with his fingers wiggling in front of this poorly focused eyes. He seemingly paid no attention to the therapist, who sat silently and attempted to grasp any possible meaning from his behavior. In the third session, the therapist began to sense that the empty outer shell of A's mannerisms, behavior, and minimal singsong vocalizations surrounded an inner perceptual experience that he was either unwilling or unable to communicate. The therapist stated that, for himself, fingers were a vehicle for reaching and touching the outer world, and in watching *A*, he sensed that *A* was admonishing his fingers to prevent them from being drawn into exploring that world. *A* was seemingly unaffected by this communication by the therapist and continued what appeared to be aimless wandering and gesturing with his fingers. The therapist became aware that he had become internally disengaged from *A* and was thinking about his next appointment. At precisely this point, *A* turned to the therapist and asked, ''Are you listening?'' What an amazing phenomenon to hear these words spoken and an amazing coincidence that it occurred at exactly the moment when the therapist was not listening.

Webster defines *coincidence* as events that occur simultaneously, take up the same place and space, and are exactly alike in shape, position, and area. Here was a therapist whose attention had strayed away from a child who immediately addressed a question in response to that occurrence. The child, amazingly, communicated verbally when he had previously been portrayed as being without communicative language. Where did these words come from? How had he developed the capacity to form them and direct them? What was the significance of this striking event?

It was on the basis of these three words that the therapist embarked upon a psychological journey with this 4-year-old patient in a long-term intensive therapeutic interaction. He was seen four to five times per week for 6 years, three times per week for 3 years, and weekly until he finished his therapy at age 17.

The therapist's immediate response to *A*'s question was to state that, in fact, he had not been listening, his attention had strayed, and he had been affected by a feeling of rejection by *A* of his efforts and had responded by turning away. (Much later, he spoke of this moment. He recalled the therapist's voice echoing inside of him and evoking an inner feeling of containment and safety.) *A* became somber and tentatively began to explore the therapist's chair with his fingers.

Following this initial communicative sentence, there was a long period of time in which *A* spent his sessions silently exploring other objects in the room and the therapist's body with his fingers. He periodically retreated into gesturing and posturing. He would alternately explore and retreat. A then brought two toy soldiers to his sessions. One was wounded and bandaged; another intact and upright. Nonverbally, he portrayed their interaction. The therapist responded by reflecting upon his reaction to A's play. The therapist spoke of the hurt and damage inflicted upon the soldier and the stiff and ineffective efforts of the erect soldier in addressing these wounds. The therapist verbalized his own inner feeling of being ineffective and stiff as he experienced a gap between A and himself. There was no immediate response, but the following morning A awoke very early and spoke his first communicative sentence to his parents, "Take me to ferapy." On that day, he arrived looking entirely different. His face was worn and haggard. He looked terrified. He was restless, agitated, and irritable. Periodically, he made sounds that were alternately whining and anguished. The picture was of a child being visciously bombarded by some internal process and helpless in managing the onslaught. The therapist spoke to what he sensed was occurring inside of A and, as he did, felt his own inner sense of stiffness dissolving. At this moment, A approached the therapist, at first stiff and tentative. He gradually molded himself into the lap of the therapist. This continued for several sessions. A indicated, at first, behaviorally and slowly with monosyllabic verbalizations, that the therapist's voice was too loud or that the lights were too bright or that the surrounding noises of the street were too intense. Everything hurt. The therapist found a way to gently hold A, turned out the lights, and drew the shades to diminish the noise level. During this period of time, A was sleepless and appeared to be in a constant state of terror. He spent many sessions in the arms of the therapist, with the therapist either silent or softly talking. The therapist remembered the earlier play with the two soldiers and spoke of the impact of outer and inner stimuli and of A's need for buffering and containment. There were several sessions where A simply slept the entire time. He then slowly began to communicate verbally. He initially described the "Make-A-Dos" and the "Big Black Pops." The Make-A-Dos were fun-loving figures but readily became angry, enlarged, and unmanageable.

The Big Black Pops were shadowy, threatening, and had to be avoided.

B was a small, frail 11-year-old boy. His frailty was accentuated by his stiff-legged manner of walking and stilted, carefully controlled speech pattern. He chose his words carefully and deliberately, with pauses between each word. His voice quality was soft, abrupt, and robotlike. Throughout his childhood, he had been fearful, easily intimidated, and unable to function in school settings. He was brought to the therapist after a period of 6 months during which he had become profoundly withdrawn and retreated into his own room. B resisted coming to the first session but quickly agreed with the therapist that he appeared to have many inner obstacles that were affecting him and that it would require a lot of work to undo them. Sessions were arranged three times per week in response to B's association to how he learned about computers. He would seek help and then need a day or two by himself to try it out. Then he was ready for more. This derivative association to the question of meeting was the only communication of this nature during the early sessions. B submissively came to his appointments and spoke only in monotonous cliches, which took the form of reporting a daily activity or event. The sessions were experienced by the therapist as lifeless and devoid of direction, and he felt an increasing sense of frustration. B then began to talk about the computers he was interested in. They could be developed to such a degree that they could eventually control the people who made them. The people who programmed them would go on thinking they were in charge, but the computer would use all the programmed information to control the programmer. This reminded him of R2D2, the robot in *Star Wars*. He appeared friendly and helpful, but B thought he was putting everyone on. He was really teasing them. That was his way of being in charge. The therapist then stated, "I have felt controlled and trapped by what has been occurring between us. I have contributed to it by continuing to try to gain some superficial understanding of your words and actions rather than sharing with you my inner sense of being teased, put on, and being controlled."

The entire quality of the interaction changed. B's immediate response was to appear stunned and to draw back with a look of hurt and confusion. He quietly spoke of how frightened he was and how much he was trying to communicate with the therapist. He felt very hurt that the therapist saw his efforts as being controlling and teasing. His voice was no longer hesitant, and he spoke with feeling for the first time.

B arrived at the following session with a determined look on his face and proceeded to what at first seemed to be an effort to move and rearrange the furniture in the room. The therapist silently moved to the side as he felt an important communication was occurring. The therapist implicitly encouraged the patient to continue. B turned all of the furniture in the room upside down and placed himself in a chair so that he was covered completely. The therapist stated that he thought B was showing him in actions his response to what had been said the previous session. After a short silence, B began to talk from beneath the chair. He had suddenly remembered an incident when he was 4 years old and was hiding under a table in exactly the position he was in now. His mother had been walking by, and he had reached out and tripped her. At the time he felt anger, mischievousness, and a sense of mastery. His mother fell, hurt herself, got up in a rage, and attacked him for his actions. The patient felt completely crushed and shattered. It felt to B like this event had been a crucial turning point in his life. From that point on, he had lost all feeling of fun and spontaneity. He became contained and fearful and constantly carried a mental image of an attacking voice that made any spontaneous feeling a source of danger. He also spoke of the despair he lived with: that any expression of emotion would drive others away, leaving him totally abandoned. The therapist stated that he had attacked B with his voice and that it must have reminded him of that inner attack. B was silent and remembered how he often retreated to his room silently-hoping someone would enter. One day his father burst into the room, which frightened him at first because he was startled and feared an attack. B was surprised that his father had entered in order to talk with him. He then thought of the many times in school when he had been bored, how much he wished he could be mischievous and play tricks on his teachers. He had always been too afraid. B then began to animatedly fantasy the many ways he could make fun of and tease people by caricaturing their mannerisms. He then made a comment as to how warm and sunny the day was.

The Effect of Empathic Responsiveness and
Empathic Failures upon Unconscious Perceptions

In these clinical examples, the therapist's acknowledgment of the patient's unconscious perceptions evoked an inner sense of containment. Empathic responsiveness in a therapeutic interaction requires validation by the patient's unconscious perceptions. A lapse or failure in the empathy of the therapist is unconsciously perceived by the patient, and the resulting interaction demands a defensive adaptation. Until the therapist can identify the source of that failure and rectify it, the interaction remains a stimulus to be defended against. It is only when the patient's unconscious perceptions are validated by the therapist that a process of inner exploration and inner integration can take place.

In the initial period with A, it was difficult to determine the presence or absence of empathic responsiveness. A reacted in a way that offered the therapist little evidence as to how he was being perceived. The therapist's attention was focused on A, and his thoughts were occupied with the interaction. The therapist's unconscious perception was of a child's wanting to reach out and fighting against that wish. The therapist communicated his perception to A and when it seemingly was ignored, the therapist reacted by withdrawing his attention. An empathic failure ensued that immediately prompted A's question, "Are you listening?" The therapist became aware of his lapse and the reasons for it, acknowledged A's unconscious perception, and A responded by communicating more freely in his exploratory behavior. Much later he described this moment as one in which he felt safe and contained. Later A was able to communicate his conconscious perception of the therapist as stiff and ineffective. The therapist's validation of this perception was followed by A's relinquishing his autistic defenses. The therapist, with A's participation, lost his stiffness and was capable of once again establishing an empathically responsive interaction. The result was in the emergence of a communicative process.

With B, a background of empathic responsiveness was initiated with the establishment of the frequency of sessions. The therapist was unconsciously perceiving B's efforts to control the relationship but was reacting defensively to that perception. The consequence for the therapist was a mounting sense of frustration and blindness to the underlying significance of this quality in the interaction. *B* derivatively communicated his unconscious perception of the controlled therapist. The therapist validated *B*'s perception, but his frustration and blindness led to an empathic failure that was manifested in an attack upon *B*'s attitude. This elicited in *B* the memory of an attack that was a parallel of the therapeutic interaction. The therapist's validation of *B*'s unconscious perception reminded *B* of his wish to be reached and was associated with an inner sense of the return of his spontaneity on a background of containment. This was expressed in his delight in the idea of mimicking authorities and sudden awareness of the warmth and brightness of the day.

The manner in which an interaction is perceived is largely determined by the development of the individual, the background relationship already established, and the therapist's interventions. When the therapist recognized the value of *A* and *B*'s unconscious perceptions, it evoked a feeling of safety. This provided a background that facilitated the emergence of psychic contents that were reactively available and unconsciously determined. In order to understand such phenomena, it is important to develop metapsychological constructs that can portray the role of perception in development and of the role of unconscious perceptions in adaptive interactions. The pathway by which a stimulus that is outside of the self can be included within the self needs to be delineated. The therapeutic interaction involves an experience outside of the self that is enhancing or hurtful to, and is included in, the processes and functions operating within the self. It is thereby essential to have a definition of the self that can be traced to its very beginnings.

The Nuclear Self—A Definition

Any definition of the early processes at the foundation of self-experience, of necessity, is highly speculative. The complex psychological experiences of later periods of development have a developmental line. A conceptual framework that is useful must broaden our view of what is observable, though it is drawn from abstractions of experiences that are not observable. Body ego experiences are at the base of all mental productions. The most advanced experiences of identity, autonomy, and separateness have a body ego experience at their foundation. This implies that the newborn infant, in a nuclear state, has a non-object-related core of perceptual activity. The activity of these primitive processes of perception leaves a body ego experience that evolves into more advanced expressions of individual separateness.

I will define the self as determined by the activity of the perceptual processes. The nuclear self is manifested with the dawning of the functions of perception. This first occurs during intrauterine life and is profoundly influenced by the surrounding maternal environment. Winnicott (1958), in developing the concept of *holding*, and Balint (1963), the concept of *primary love*, allude to this intrauterine model as a reflection of the maternal figure's influence on the earliest experiences that provide definition to the nuclear self. Bion's (1968) metaphor of the container and the contained makes direct reference to this model.

These anlagen of autonomously functioning perceptual processes, influenced by the stimuli of the surrounding maternal environment and the stimuli of biophysiology, exert their effects. The manner in which they function delineates a boundary for the nuclear self. The boundary is limited by the nature of these anlagen and by the ego's capacity to represent the perceptions. The beginning development of an ego is founded upon these bodily experiences and the perceptions of them. For this reason, the original ego is a body ego. Each perceptual experience stimulates responses from two distinct and sequential areas of mental activities. The first area of activity can be referred to as *representation*, in which the stimulus upon entering the field of perception is registered as a mental impression. The force of the stimulus impacts upon the perceptual processes in such a way as to leave an impresson that is registered and remains. This is followed by the second area of mental activity, referred to as *organization*, in which these mental impressions are organized into an identifiable unit.

Perceptual experiences fall into two general categories, each of which have differing degrees of impact on the representational and organizational functions. One group of perceptual experiences emanate from the sensory modalities of touch, temperature, smell, and taste that are closer to the immediacy of bodily processes. These close receptors have a high capacity to represent stimuli and a low capacity to organize these stimuli as emanating from a given source. Thus, touch, temperature, smell, and taste will be the most represented (and in those body geographic zones most highly innervated). The other group of perceptual experiences emanate from the sensory modalities of hearing and sight, which are more distant from the immediacy of bodily processses. These distant receptors have a low-representational and a high-organizational capacity. Hearing and sight will be least represented, and in the earliest phases of development, their organization influence will be very limited. The representations of the activities of these primitive perceptual processes will gradually coalese according to the nature of the stimuli and capacities of the child. These are the beginnings of psychic structuralization and are forming the varied aspects of what will become a self-representational system. These self-representations form within the boundaries of the nuclear self and reflect differing responses to varied stimuli. Advances in development, together with the maturation of the autonomous ego funcitons, will consolidate these part self-representations into a totality. This process will be accelerated as the distant perceptual processes exert their organizational influence. Spitz (1955) and Hoffer (1952) have stressed this organizing influence of the perceptual processes.

The manner in which a given body ego experience is represented varies according to the particular locale at which the activity of perception takes place. This is important for the understanding of those body ego experiences upon which the foundation of unconscious perceptions are based. Unconscious perceptions are manifested either by derivatives that express their activity or by the internal state reactively evoked by a stimulus. The unconscious perception of an interaction is initiated by a stimulus at the periphery (the point of contact with the external world). This has a different effect than a stimulus at the interior (the point of contact with the impact of biophysiology). This difference was manifested in *A* in the representations of the Make-A-Dos and the Big Black Pops. The Make-A-Dos were instinctual in nature and reflected the effects of contact with the demands of biophysiology. They were fluctuating in their instinctual qualities and reflective of bodily processes. The Big Black Pops were prohibitive in nature and reflected the effects of contact with the impinging stimuli of the external world. The impinging qualities of the Make-A-Dos were overstimulating. The impinging qualities of the Big Black Pops were attacking and patterned after an object in the external world. The unconscious perception of an interaction registers the effects of a stimulus at the periphery.

Representation also depends upon the nature of the stimulus and the state of the mental mechanisms available for its registration. Voluntary bodily processes are more definitive and capable of being perceived by the early body ego. Involuntary bodily processes are registered with a diminished intensity or not at all. The consolidation of the part self-representations into an entity is accompanied by the concurrent integration of the perceptual processes. Some degree of integration is necessary for unconscious perceptions to be functional. Consensual validation refers to the integration of perceptual processes and results in the dual functions of representation and organization becoming available within all perceptual modalities. Visual and auditory stimuli can then affect other sensory modalities and vice versa. The capacity to register and express the effects of unconscious perceptions is dependent upon this developmental step of establishing consensual validation.

The degree of intensity of perceptual contact with the external world depends on its nature and impact. Contacts of lesser intensity or with little evocative connection to the representations of bodily processes have little effect. Contacts of great intensity or with a high degree of evocative connection to the representations of bodily processes have a great impact. Thus, with *A*, the therapist's lapse of attention was immediately reacted to and unconsciously perceived as a potential threat. There was an evocative connection to the experience of abandonment and its profound effect on bodily processes. This quality of a lapse in attention would have affected *B* with little impact because it did not establish such an evocative connection. With *B*, the therapist's intervention was tinged with frustration and had a powerful impact on his unconscious perceptions. There was an evocative link to the screen memory of trauma that made him exquisitely unconsciously perceptive of these interactional qualities.

*The Background Object of Primary Identification and
Its Significance for the Nuclear Self*

The first perceptual contact with the external world is intrauterine. The primordial nuclear self registers the containing, regulating aspect of a primary identification with the buffering, physiological, and metabolizing function of the intrauterine maternal environment. This forms a representation in the nuclear self, excellently named the "background object of primary identification," by Grotstein (1981). The background object of primary identificaiton is expanded through the containing, regulating interactions with the mothering external object in postuterine life. This is the representation of a body ego experience that allows the establishment of a psychological symbiosis. The mothering figure's psychological containment and the psychological metabolism of the infant's emotional interchanges are dependent upon the presence of this body ego experience. The background object of primary identification is the representation of a body ego experience of contact with the intrauterine environment, is present at birth, and establishes a foundation for the introjection and representation of the activities of perception in interactions with the external world. A mental vehicle is available by which a stimulus emanating from outside of the self, through its evocative connection to a structure inside of the self, can be included and contribute to its expansion. When *A* was verbally uncommunicative, much of the understanding of the interaction depended upon the inferences of the therapist. *A* behaviorally explored both the room and the therapist with his fingers. He alternately explored and retreated. His behavior shifted to play with two soldiers that appeared to the therapist to exactly parallel how the therapist was experiencing the interaction. He saw *A* as being wounded and damaged and himself as being stiff and ineffective in helping him. The therapist's realization of his stiffness had implicit in it the potential for undoing it. The therapist was offering his help to *A* and also indicating his openness to be helped. This quality parallels the mutuality that is involved in symbiotic interactions. The therapist's communication had a profound effect on *A*. He became verbally communicative, and stimuli that he had previously seemed oblivious to were experienced as impinging. *A* molded himself to the therapist; the therapist felt his stiffness dissolve, and the therapist was able to buffer *A* from the traumatic impact of these impinging stimuli. *A* spent many sessions molding himself physically and psychologically to the containing activities of the therapist. These interactions were empathic to, and resonant with, *A*'s inner needs. They provided buffering and did not elicit defensive reactions to impingement. During this period of time, *A* appeared to be in a state of fusion with the therapist. He was soothed and comforted in the arms of the therapist and had shifted from the position of warding off the stimuli of the external world, which at first had been so powerful and impinging. This was reminiscent of Mahler *et al.*'s (1975) description of the psychological symbiosis of early development. This state of lack of differentiation could only evolve in *A* when the therapist was empathically responsive with consistency over time. This was consonant with the idea that a psychological symbiosis is a developmental advance and only evolves when the interaction is empathic to and resonant with inner need; that is, the state of lack of differentiation that characterizes a symbiosis evolves out of an empathic interaction and is not present from the outset. Further, for this psychological symbiosis to transpire, there must be an already-existent body ego experience that has been represented to serve as a foundation. This body ego experience is the representation of the background object of primary identification. In *A*, the degree of fragmentation in his mental representations was reflective of the deficiency in the representations of the background object. This seemed to give emphasis to the process by which new self- and object representations are formed and expanded upon. That is, the background object of primary identification is the body ego experience upon which symbiotic interactions are dependent, and these symbiotic interactions are necessary for the building of new self- and object representations.

Qualities of Goodness and Badness and Their Representation in the Nuclear Self

Goodness refers to the representation of experiences that have no necessity for defense. *Badness* refers to the representation of experiences that require defense. The part self-representations will be united into a whole, with the varied qualities of goodness and badness consolidating into separate entities. Differing facets of good experience and bad experience unite, though lines of cleavage are identifiable when the self-representations are under stress.

The Part Self-Representations of Goodness

A whole good self-representation is formed from the body ego experience of the various facets of goodness; there are three facets:

1. First is the background object of primary identification. the primordial nuclear self registers contact with the containing, regulating, metabolizing aspect of the maternal environment without the need for defense.

2. Second is the instinctual activity that is perceived and represented without the need for defense. At this early stage of development, the body ego experiences involve libidinal zones associated with orality. The totality of these perceptual experiences encompasses additional dimensions. The object in the external world provides empathic contact, whereby the infant has the body ego experience of gratification of an instinctual demand. The empathic responses of the external object eventuate in a multiplicity of body ego experiences. Those aspects of the interaction that are optimally gratifying provide body ego experiences that are represented as the good instinctual facet of the self. The nature of the mental impressions defines the instinctual activity, and the emphasis is on body geographic zones associated with orality.

3. Third is the representation of the activity of the autonomous ego functions. The infant, in its nuclear condition, has the seeds of what will become a conflict-free sphere of the ego and of autonomous functions in a primitive form. These ego functions are not yet structuralized, effective, or readily accessible. They are present in a state of readiness to be evoked and amplified in response to appropriate stimuli. The optimally frustrating element of empathic responsiveness is necessary to both evoke and support these functions. The empathic object in the external world is not only empathic with the instinctual demands of the infant but with the anlage of the infant's autonomous functioning. An empathic mother will respond to the beginnings of function barely

visible within the infant. These functions are amplified by her empathic activity. The body ego experience within the infant is one of resonance and connection. An object outside of the self amplifies a function within the self. This quality of interaction has awakened the activity of the ego. Optimal gratification in an interaction depends upon qualities of optimal frustration. It is essential for the empathically responding object in the external world to be sensitive to when the developing infant can wait for the gratification of instinctual demands. The period of waiting is occupied with the exercise of the autonomous ego functions. These functions are exercised and utilized to participate in the building of psychic structure and to engage in defensive and integrative activities. Hartmann (1939), in calling attention to this crucial aspect of early development, expanded psychoanalytic metapsychology to include the psychology of the ego. Psychic representation is initiated with the dawning of perceptual activity *in utero* and manifested by the background object of primary identification. This would also indicate the existence of primitive defensive activity. Perception, being a function of the ego, would of necessity have at least some reactive discriminatory capacity. *A* had withdrawn from the stimuli of the external world very early in his development and yet continued to represent the stimuli of the internal world of biophysiologic demand. His withdrawal was not complete in that he was extremely reactive to the stimuli of interactions with objects in the external world, and these interactions influenced the part self- and part object representations that had formed. Ego functions engaged in defense were seemingly present from the outset. The absence of optimally gratifying and optimally frustrating interactions had not provided sufficient representation and consolidation of the qualities of goodness for these ego functions to participate in the building of psychic structure. The qualities of goodness that were present in *A* were only mobilized in the presence of a background of empathy that lapsed. This was expressed in his original question, ''Are you listening?'' This indicated the existence of a capacity to momentarily organize the qualities of goodness into a whole, and specifically in response to an empathic failure. These organized qualities of goodness were not consistently present at the point of contact with the external world. It seemed to suggest that these qualities of goodness had organized and were responsive to the need for defense.

Thus the varied facets of goodness represented in the self are those of the representation of the background object of primary identification, of instinctual gratification, and of the activity of the autonomous ego functions. At the onset of development, the facets of goodness have to be represented at the interior to allow the processes of internalization and structure building to take place. The foundation of unconscious perceptions is based on these body ego experiences. The qualities of a therapeutic interaction will be evocative to these developmental structures. The interventions of a therapist, when empathic to the unconscious communications of a patient, will then be validated by derivative expressions of these qualities of goodness. This will be particularly true of the manner in which the therapist manages the framework of the therapy. The qualities of containment, regulation, optimal gratification, and optimal frustration are most powerfully communicated in this dimension. Langs (1977) has consistently drawn attention to this frequently overlooked aspect of the therapeutic interaction.

The Part Self-Representations of Badness

A whole bad self-representation is formed from the body ego experience of the various facets of badness; there are three:

1. One facet is instinctual. Libidinal activity is on a continuum of intensity. The overstimulating dimension of that continuum mobilizes a defensive response. The aggressive qualities of instinctual demand, when contained and regulated, are differentiating in their effects. The primitive state of the union of the libidinal drives, which are beyond the bounds of phase specificity and the aggressive drives requiring defense, are represented as greed in the bad self when the focus is on the erotogenic zones of orality.

2. The second facet consists of the body ego experiences of reacting to impingement. When stimuli encroach upon or strike the perceptual processes with great force or intensity, they mobilize the defensive capacities of the ego. These are expressed in mechanisms of fight, flight, and/or withdrawal.

3. The third facet represented as a part of the bad self consists of the body ego experiences of sensory deprivations. The virtual impossibility of providing a totally empathic environment means that there is always a sector of sensory deprivation.

Initially, these qualities of badness are represented at the periphery (the point of perceptual contact with the external world), serve a protective function, and facilitate differentiation. Bad qualities all involve responses that are modeled after the reactions to impingement. That is, there is a fight against, a fleeing from, or a withdrawal from the source of stimulation.

The representations of good self-experience are forming at the interior (the point of perceptual contact with the demands of biophysiology and the effects of the functioning of bodily processes). These good self-representations modulate the potential traumatic effect of the intensity of the perceptual impact of biophysiologic demands and the effects of bodily processes. The experience of optimal gratification is represented when the background object of primary identication is amplified by the empathic activities of the external environment. This movement toward the inclusion of a source of external stimulation expresses the binding function of libido. A state of lack of differentiation is a prerequisite for this psychological symbiotic interaction to occur and is necessary to enable the building of new structure. The bad self-representations, forming at the periphery, offer some balance to that lack of differentiation. When the stimuli of interactions with the external world possess overstimulating, impinging, or depriving qualities, they are immediately evocative of the defensive responsiveness of the represented qualities of badness. Although the whole bad and whole good self-representations are consolidating as separate entities, there is a line of connection between them. The representation of instinctual activity in the good self shades into the representation of instinctual activity in the bad self, maintaining a line of continuity.

The Consolidation of the Representations of the Self and the Development of Consensual Validation

Initially, the three facets of the whole good self are represented separately. The source of instinctual gratification, the source of the background object of primary identification, and the source of the body ego experience of the exercise of autonomous ego functions are different. There is some overlapping, but there is sufficient difference to form lines of cleavage. The three facets of the whole bad self are also repesented separately. The source of instinctual overstimulation, the source of the reactions to impingment, and the source of sensory deprivations are sufficiently different to form lines of cleavage. The integration and maturation of all perceptual processes occur concurrently with the consolidation of the part self-representations into a whole.

The earliest boundaries of the self are body ego experiences represented primarily as a result of the activity of the near receptors of touch, taste, and smell and only minimally through the distant receptors of hearing and sight. These near receptors have a limited organizing capacity and a strong ability to be represented. The distant receptors have a limited representational capacity and a strong capacity for organization. Self-representations and the object impressions form within these boundaries to make up the totality of the self. The maturation of perceptual functions is interrelated with the consolidation of the self-representations and increases the availability of the organizing function of the distant receptors. An interdependent relationship is established in which the consolidation of the self-representations into a whole and the integration of the near and far receptors operate in concert with each other. The various perceptual modalities then function in unison. The manner in which unconscious perceptions are activated and manifest their functioning is directly proportional to the degree of integration of the organizing and representational functions of perceptual processes. In this fashion, emotional nuances in an interaction can be perceived through one perceptual modality and evoke a total response. The boundaries of the self gradually become more delineated and organized as the representational and organizational functions achieve continuity with all perceptual processes. Consensual validation is thus possible. A, even with the state of fragmentation that dominated his psychic functioning, was capable of a transient experience of inner consolidation of the whole good self. It was evoked by the unconscious perception of a lapse in the therapist's attention. Consensual validation had to be functional, at least momentarily, to accomplish this perceptual act. Qualities of goodness were so insufficiently represented in A, that this degree of consolidation could not be maintained. Consensual validation means that both functions of representation and organization become available to all perceptual modalities.

Splitting as a Translocation of Perception

Unconscious perceptions are a reflection of the effects of a stimulus occurring at one locale and having continuity with its representation to another sector of the personality. It seems important to try to formulate the original developmental processes that have embodied this quality of perception. Kernberg (1980) has described splitting as self, object, affect units organized and split off from each other according to their good and bad qualities. He did not give any indication of how this evolves. I have had the experience with a small group of children, such as *A*, where it was possible for me to participate in interactions that eventuated in the form of new representational structures. From the manner in which this transpired, I have attempted to abstract a concept that may illuminate these early processes. It appeared to me that the mechanism of splitting involved a translocation of perception that is, a process in which the representation of a stimulus occurred away from its source. The body ego experience of this process could serve as a foundation for the expression of unconscious perceptions. (It could also be a foundation for the functioning of repression proper. *Primal repression* refers to the interface of the realm of biology, making demands, with the mental realm of representation. *Repression proper* is an active mental process in which perceptual attention is directed away from one sequence of psychic events and attracted to another.)

Stimulation is continuously present at the interior from the effects of biophysiology. In addition, stimulation is present at the periphery from the effects of interactions with the external world. The impact of biophysiology is variable and dependent upon the manner in which its demands can be represented. The perceptual processes register a certain amount as phase-specific instinctual gratification. The containing, ministrating interactions with the external world provide a body ego experience of stability evocative of the background object of primary identification and enhance these representations of good instinctual experience. The optimally frustrating qualities of an empathic interaction amplify the autonomous ego functions. These part good self-representations consolidate into a whole at the interior. The point of perceptual contact, however, is at the periphery.

The intensity of the biophysiologic impact is such that a certain amount is overstimulating and potentially traumatic. The quality of the impact is that of an impingement. This aspect of biophysiologic demand mobilizes defense and is represented as the instinctual aspect of the bad self. The body ego experiences that result from the impinging, nonempathic interactions with the object in the external world are represented at the periphery. These stimulate reactions to impingement and are also represented as a facet of the bad self. These qualities of badness are consolidating at the periphery. The impinging quality of the demands of biophysiology is evocative of the impinging qualities of the interactions with the object in the external world. These part bad self-representations, along with the representations of sensory deprivation, organize into a whole at the periphery. Thus the developing whole bad self-representations are forming at the periphery, though the instinctual stimulus is at the interior.

It is this translocation of perception, in which the representation of a stimulus occurs away from its source, that I am postulating as the basis for the mechanism of splitting. this mechanism furthers the developmental process, serves a protective function, and evolves as the major defensive activity of the primitively organized ego.

The Self with Object Qualities and the Object with Self-Qualities

The continuum of biophysiologic demands stimulate body ego experiences of such a varying quality that they are represented as separate facets within the totality of the self. The continuum ranges from body ego experiences represented as phase-specific instinctual gratification in the good self, to body ego experiences (of overstimulation with qualities of an impingement) represented as the instinctual aspect of the bad self. The continuum extends to body ego experiences that are of such an intensity that they cannot be represented as aspects of the self. They are, however, leaving mental impressions of an impact that is impinging and instinctual. These impressions, in not being included within the self-representations, have the independent qualities of an object. They are forming as bad instinctual object impressions that ultimately will become more organized and represented as the bad instinctual aspect of the object. The continuum also extends to that dimension of biophysiologic demand that cannot be perceived and represented. It is this aspect of the continuum that is present within the organism but is independent of the self. With advances in development, the capacity for instinctual representation increases, the continuum shifts, and more is included within the self. This continuum provides the original body ego experience by which stimuli originating outside of the self (yet within the organism) are included within the self. I have named this continuum, as mentioned before, "the self with object qualities." The manner in which the Make-A-Dos were represented in *A* captured the qualities of this continuum. These instinctual representations were on a continuum from being fun loving and represented as an aspect of the good self, to being irritable and impinging and represented as an aspect of the bad self, to being ominous, frightening, and represented with the qualities of a bad instinctual object. It is this end of the continuum that I consider to be the portal of entry of instinctual demand. An empathically responsive interaction and its associated experience of containment should have the effect of including more of this continuum within the realm of self-representation. Conversely, a nonempathic interaction would have the effect of intensifying the threat of this continuum. Melanie Klein (1955) described the oedipal conflict as originating very early in development. This concept emerged from the observation of these object impressions with instinctual qualities that were so intense and potentially disruptive. Balint (1968), in his concept of the basic fault, was noticing the influence of this continuum. Bion (1968) described it as the psychotic sector of the personality. It is the body ego experience that ultimately forms the basis for object-related perceptions; that is, the capacity for perceiving the object as having independent objects of its own (a necessary component of the oedipal conflict). In that sense, it can be seen as a precursor of the oedipal conflict.

The body ego experiences of empathic contact with an external object, together with the primitive state of the organizational functions of the perceptual processes, combine to facilitate a psychological symbiosis. Mental representations of a good self grow and consolidate as a result of these empathic experiences. Interactions with an external object are also on a continuum. In the state of lack of differentiation, those aspects that are optimally gratifying have self-qualities. The aspects of the continuum that are optimally frustrating have qualities of prohibition, and these prohibitive aspects shade into the area of being unempathic and impinging. As I said previously, I have named this continuum "the object with self qualities." The ongoing interactions with the object with self-qualities are registered and advance the expanding representations of the good and bad selves. These interactions are also forming mental impressions, of a poorly differentiated quality, that later will evolve into an object representational system. The self with object qualities and the object with self-qualities are providing the necessary body ego experiences by which stimuli originating outside of the self can be included, through representation, within the self.

Discussion

A's psychic functioning manifested the effects of severe pathological distortions in his development. The therapist attempted to establish a surrounding external environment that would be evocative to whatever good self-representations were available. The therapist saw his task as one of offering optimal gratification in the form of empathic responsiveness to expressions of unconscious communication, optimal frustration in the form of abstaining from participation in the reinforcement of pathological defenses, and the qualities of a transitional object in the form of implicitly encouraging A to utilize the relationship in whatever way that was dictated by his development. The therapist was offering an interaction with the characteristics of being nonimpinging and of be-

ing responsive to the unconscious communications expressed in
A's behavior. Initially, *A* seemed not to respond. A lapse in the
therapist's empathic responsiveness instigated a momentary level
of organization in *A* that permitted an integrated, interactively
communicative expression. *A* had been unconsciously perceptive
of the therapist's lapse in attention. It required the presence of consensual validation for this perceptual act to have taken place. This
would imply that there had been a momentary consolidation of
the part self-representations into a unity. *A*'s unconscious perception of the therapist's defensiveness was again manifested in his
play with the soldiers. His play seemed to mirror the therapist's
stiffness. When the therapist validated *A*'s unconscious perception, first by acknowledging the fact that he had disengaged from
A and later by acknowledging the stiffness and ineffectiveness he
felt, it resulted in a dramatic shift in *A*'s communicative behavior.
The organizing influence of the background object of primary identification became manifest. In the first instance, *A* felt contained
and openly engaged in an exploration of the therapist. In the second instance, *A* relinquished his autistic posture, molded to the
therapist, and began to verbally communicate his inner experiences. The therapist's acknowledgment of *A*'s unconscious
perception was accompanied, in both instances, by a change in the
therapist's attitude. *A* had made the therapist aware of the lapse
in empathy, but it was essential that the therapist see the source
of it in himself and effect a change.

   B manifested pathology with a higher level of organization. He
was capable of direct verbal communication and of associating
derivatively to the meaning of the interaction. Initially, *B* was fearful of the new relationship and resisted coming. He was immediately receptive to the therapist's recognition of his inner turmoil.
B felt unconsciously understood when the frequency of sessions
was determined by his derivative association. In this way, *B* was
programming the therapist. *B*, in his submissive attitude, communicated his experience of being controlled. The therapist unconsciously perceived this quality in the interaction and reacted
defensively to being seen as a controlling figure. In so doing, he
was no longer responding empathically. The therapist then communicated his feeling of being controlled. However, in being un-
aware of its source, the therapist was implying that the motive was

within *B*. The background of empathy that had been established was traumatically ruptured and mobilized *B*'s resources. He responded by revealing the manner in which the therapist's intervention was experienced. It was a parallel repetition of a developmental trauma. The therapist finally grasped the part he had played in creating the rupture and was able to validate *B*'s unconscious perception. The result was in the emergence of mischievousness and self-assertiveness. *B*'s lively fantasies of caricaturing people's mannerisms reflected the presence of instinctual activities that had previously been repressed. His derivative association to his fear of his father's bursting into his room and surprise that he had wanted to talk with him reflected upon his unconscious perception of the change in the therapist's attitude.

During the earliest phases in development, instinctual demands are registered in an ongoing interrelationship with the physiologically buffering contact with the intrauterine environment. The representation of this experience froms a background that fosters the expansion of all further mental growth. This background object of primary identification reflects the interrelationship of inner demand and outer metabolic response and establishes a body ego experience by which a stimulus outside of the self (defined by the activity of perceptual processes) is included within the self. This is the original body ego experience at the foundation of the psychological symbiosis of postuterine life. It underlies the pathway by which the qualities of an interaction are unconsciously perceived. When the containing, metabolizing effects of the background object of primary identification are actively functional, the interpretive activity of the therapist can be included within the self. When the therapist's activities are in response to the unconscious experiences of the patient, this representation is evoked, and there is no necessity for adaptive and defensive reactions to impingement to be mobilized.

CHAPTER 2

The Qualities of Perceptual Experience and Object Impressions
The Self- and Object Representational Systems

Introduction

In my efforts to understand the significance of the effect of the therapist in the therapeutic interaction, several qualities of experience stood out. I noticed that when I was sensitively in tune with my patient's inner unconscious experience, the patient's experience was not one of interacting with a unidimensional object. On those occasions, the patients seemed to perceive me as a more complete multidimensional figure. In addition, at those moments, my manner of interacting had the combined qualities of a whole good object. That is, there was an optimal level of gratification associated with an optimal level of frustration, appropriate to the therapeutic interaction, that occurred in a matrix of an ability to function in the manner of a transitional object. I did not have to defend myself against the interactional pressures exerted upon me and could allow the patient to experience me in his or her own individual way without my opposition. I also noticed that when I was reacting defensively to the interaction, although I maintained a myriad and variety of internal experiences and responses, my patient experienced me as a unidimensional part object. This was particularly evident in those patients who were more primitively organized. It was more subtly present in those who had attained higher levels of personality organization. The recognition in my more primitive patients made me aware of the subtleties. I also became aware that my patient was a participant in eliciting in me exactly those qualities that would highlight a particular aspect of a bad object's influence.

With autistic children, the therapeutic interaction functioned to consolidate their representational world and revealed the manner by which mental representations and perceptual processes were interrelated in their evolution. It also shed light upon the effects of an external object and the qualities of experience that facilitated new structure building or obviated against it. Unconscious perceptions were intimately linked to body ego experiences, so that when a healthy, well-contained interaction was offered, the patient's unconscious perceptions emerged as undistorted. Although the way I was perceived was strongly influenced by their developmental experience with external objects, pathological distortions only surfaced in response to pathology in the interaction. It was only within a healthy framework that the work of integrating pathological contents could take place.

I will attempt to describe the manner in which a system of object representations is built up within the boundaries of the self. The varying effects of stimuli that are independent of the self leave mental impressions that serve as a foundation for the representation of an object. Every self-representation has such a counterpart that reflects the manner in which the underlying body ego experience has occurred. The interrelationship forms the groundwork for continuing self-expansion and influences the perceptual processes that create them.

Clinical Material

A slowly began to talk, first from the position of being cradled by the therapist. He gradually shifted from that position to physically moving around the room. At times he was contained, and at times he was agitated. He talked about the internal creatures that assaulted him and the occasional figures that comforted him. When he spoke of the assaulting figures, his agitation mounted.

When he spoke of the comforting figures, he appeared contained. When he spoke of mischievous and fun-loving creatures, he smiled. Although he had exhibited a variety of facial expressions, this was the first time he had smiled. His communicative speech was soft, with many words difficult for the therapist to understand. The names he assigned to the mental objects that populated his mind were spoken very clearly. His descriptions were accentuated by his whole manner and captured the particular function and effect that these objects had upon him.

The Make-A-Dos, as mentioned, were the most variable. They changed from mischievous, fun-loving, impish characters, to angry, hostile, troublesome creatures, to very frightening, provocative, seductive figures who escalated in size. They were associated with an inner feeling of overexcitement and irritability. The name of these figures shed some light on his lifelong episodes of severe constipation. There had been two occasions earlier in his life that required hospitalization when he had not had a bowel movement for as long as a month. The Make-A-Dos emerged as creatures with instinctual qualities that ranged from goodness to badness to an ominous quality. The Big Black Pops were dark, partly hidden sticklike figures. They were extremely explosive, prohibitive, and frightening. His whole being was immobilized when he felt their inner presence. The prohibitive qualities were unmistakable. "The Big Pain" was a maternal figure who suffered intensely at the expression of any suffering. Everything that involved conflict or psychic pain, in turn, hurt The Big Pain. This figure was constantly whining and commiserating. "Pa-Ba" was an undernourished, undeveloped, undefined, deprived, and helpless infant. Interspersed with A's description of these inner objects was the gradual emergence of the soldier. This figure varied from being firm, steadfast, reality bound, and insisting on performance, to being soft, understanding, and warmly responsive. In the presence of the soldier, there was always an aura of containment.

C began psychotherapy at the age of 7, when his surrounding environment felt totally inadequate in dealing with his inability or refusal to complete any task. His wild clowning and disruptive behavior alternated with periods of profound depression and explosive temper tantrums, usually in response to a demand or frustrating task. The overall picture was of a controlling, greedy, highly manipulative child, who managed to engage one adult after another into feeling sorry for him and taking care of him. Initially, he was seen one time per week. The idea of meeting more frequently evoked an intense negative reaction. The first 2 years were occupied with teasing and spinning fantasies of his life, wishes, and hopes. Many of the fantasies were explosively aggressive and some highly eroticized. There were repeated efforts to engage the therapist into joining him in his manipulative, conniving plots or in the acting out of his fantasies. C would tease the therapist about his interpretive responses. The depreciatory teasing always had an element of relief. Slowly C made both himself and the therapist aware of his deep inner sense of inadequacy covered by his provocations and manipulations. A serious separation anxiety, in being addressed by the therapist, led to C's establishing his sessions three times per week. A concern with inner fragmentation was manifested in frequent nightmares and in the threat of separation from familiar objects. The sessions most difficult for C were those in which he felt empty, wordless, blocked, and restless. He appeared, at these times, like he could hardly tolerate keeping himself within the confines of the office. In his effort to deal with this anxiety, C found a plastic egg-shaped puzzle that broke down into many pieces and could be reassembled. He wanted to use it to help him become able to talk and not run from the office. The following session occurred at this point in the therapy.

C entered the office, took out the puzzle, dissembled it, and began to put it together. As he did so, he spoke of his difficulty when something did not immediately fit. He wanted to discipline himself to be able to search for and find just the right piece. The therapist responded by metaphorically relating the pieces of the puzzle to the pieces of himself. At first, C reacted with delight and elaborated the metaphor. However, as the session was ending, C stated, partly with the teasing, depreciatory qualities that characterized his reaction to interpretive efforts but also with a note of sadness and despair. "What good does it do to talk about pieces of a puzzle? What does that have to do with me?" The therapist stated that he thought it had everything to do with C, including his attempt to deal with the separation at the end of the hour, by making the therapist see and feel his despair and feel the anxiety that C experienced as his inner contents came closer to him. C remained silent for the remainder of the session and left appearing somewhat dejected.

He entered the next session, following a weekend, extremely excited and eager to talk. He had been invited to someone's house over the weekend. This is an activity he had always previously avoided. On this occasion he decided to go. When it came time to go to sleep, he was filled with a state of panic. He felt the temptation to return to his home but decided to stay in his bed for a while. He began to think about the puzzle he had been working on in the therapist's office and of the therapist's words. He thought to himself, ''What are these pieces of myself?'' They must be the things I feel and think about. He began to allow himself to be filled with and observe what entered his mind. He thought of his interest in *Playboy* and his sexual excitement. This immediately led to a recollection of his masturbatory experiences. A tremendous feeling of shame and embarrassment filled him as he thought of it. The associative chain was interrupted by a feeling of anxiety and uncomfortable excitement. His thoughts shifted, and he recalled the sports in which he was an effective participant. He also thought of his schoolwork. It was overwhelming and frustrating. He could feel the potential that was not being realized and the frustration associated with it. As his inner feeling of inadequacy mounted, his thoughts shifted again to a favored place in the country. Here he could be with himself and feel free, contained, and soothed. This inner calmness was immediately interrupted by memories of his rage in response to the intimidating attacks of demanding teachers. These memories were either of being totally intimidated, reacting in a rage and becoming humiliated, or of his total submissive retreat. His memories moved toward his family. He recalled his mother's efforts to empathize with his suffering. At times it was quite helpful, but it was so easy for him to manipulate her by his suffering. He could make her feel guilty and get his way. He thought of his father's contempt for C's greedy behavior or inadequacies in performance, yet how much he looked for his father's curtailment. This quickly shifted to a feeling of being impinged upon by the frightening aspects of his father's anger at him. He thought of his dog, which he loved dearly, and of his overattachment to material objects. He began to realize that when he was confronted with a separation, he attached comforting qualities to some material object that would be envied by others. As his thoughts roamed to the things he was most interested in, such as fireworks and guns, and how alone he felt with those interests, he began to have an inner sensation of coming together. It reminded him of the sensation of completing a puzzle, finding the right piece, and having it click into place. The panic had dissolved. He spent the remainder of the weekend feeling himself a whole and separate person.

The Conditions for Establishing a System of Object Representations

The boundaries of the nuclear self gradually become more firmly established as the differing part self-representations coalesce into a whole. Within these boundaries, the body ego experiences of varying stimuli continue to be represented. The maturation of the perceptual processes is interrelated with the progressive developments in the self-representational system. This evolution of maturation and consolidation of the self-representations is an important precondition for the establishment of a system of object representations. Although the mental impressions of independent stimuli are present within the boundaries of the nuclear self, they have not as yet been organized into a system of representations.

Initially, the qualities of good self-experience consolidate in the interior, at the point of perceptual contact with biophysiologic demand. The containing effect of a whole good self-representation is most needed at this site, to balance the disruptive impact of those qualities of biophysiological demands that are impinging. A stimulus at the periphery of the organism, at the point of contact with the external world, has a different effect than a stimulus at the interior. This difference was manifested in A in the representations of the Make-A-Dos and the Big Black Pops. The Make-A-Dos were instinctual in nature and reflected the effects of contact with the demands of biophysiology. They were fluctuating in their instinctual qualities and reflective of bodily processes. The Big Black Pops were prohibitive in nature and reflected the effects of contact with the impingements of the external world. The impinging qualities of the Make-A-Dos were overstimulating and required defense. The impinging qualities of the Big Black Pops also required defense but were attacking in nature and patterned after an object in the external world.

The varied facets of bad self-experience are represented and coalesce at the periphery, at the point of perceptual contact with the external world. The whole bad self-representations are localized at this site where the impingements of the external world are registered, to provide a differentiating influence. The whole good self-representation forming at the interior and the whole bad self-representation forming at the periphery give expression to the mechanism of splitting. Empathic contact at the periphery resonates with the consolidating representations of the good self and draws perceptual attention and further representation at the interior (the object with self-qualities). The overstimulating aspects of instinctual demand at the interior resonate with, and draw perceptual attention and further representation to, the consolidating representations of the bad self at the periphery (the self with object qualities). The result is in the buildup of stabilized good whole self-representations at the interior. A line of continuity is maintained because the demands of biophysiology are on a continuum, which is represented as phase-specific instinctual gratification in the good self and shades into the representation of instinctual overstimulation in the bad self.

The Initial Object Impressions and Their Further Representation

The Make-A-Dos in *A* possessed differing qualities. They were represented and named, indicating that they originated from a single source of stimulation. They could be fun loving (and not require defense), threatening (and mobilize defensive responses), and ominous (and possess the attributes of a bad object). This latter aspect of instinctual representation, as a bad object, appeared to be present as an object impression with the onset of perceptual experience. It would suggest that the demands of biophysiology have the most powerful impact on the perceptual processes in the earliest stages of development. In addition, these biophysiological demands, which are on a continuum, in being represented as having differing qualities, would indicate that they are registered by perceptual processes with a high capacity for representation and a low capacity for organization. These representations act as a nidus that determines the necessity for defense and defines the qualities of goodness and badness. The continuum of biophysiologic demand is represented as the instinctual facets of the good and bad selves and of the bad object. This perspective stresses the dependence of the infant upon empathic interactions for the development of stability.

The representation of the background object of primary identification has formed from the experience of perceptual contact with the intrauterine environment. The object impression of this self-representation has the characteristics of a transitional object and fosters the development of a representational system that is separate from the system of self-representations and yet within the boundaries of the self. It is a mental impression of an object's containing influence that is separated from the self-representations and is a part of the self.

I am postulating the primordial presence of two poorly defined, poorly differentiated mental impressions of an object, each of which serves as a nidus for good and bad qualities and that will ultimately expand, develop, and elaborate into a more complex system of object representations. One, the instinctual representation of a bad object, forms at the interior (the point of perceptual contact with the demands of biophysiology). This is the nidus around which the other represented aspects of a bad object will coalesce. The other, the representation of a transitional object, forms at the periphery (the point of perceptual contact with the external world). This is the nidus around which the other represented aspects of a good object will coalesce.

Object impressions refer to the effect of a stimulus, which is independent of the self, upon the perceptual processes. These are the counterparts of the body ego experiences at the foundation of self-representations. Each facet of body ego experience has its object-impression counterpart. They evolve from interactions with the external world (and its empathic, impinging, and depriving qualities) and from contact with the demands of biology that are capable of representation. Ultimately, they will coalesce into a whole good and bad representation of an object. Body ego experiences, having a more powerful impact, necessitate a translocation of perception to enable the self-representations to consolidate. The good and bad selves are thereby represented away from the source of a stimulus. The object impressions remain at the site of a stimulus, where they are represented and consolidate.

The Representations of the Good Object

The stimuli of empathic interactions take place at the periphery, and the object impressions of these good qualities of experience consolidate at this locale to form the representation of a whole good object. There are three facets:

1. One facet is the mental impression of an object providing phase-specific instinctual gratification. The perceptual processes, gaining increasing maturation and integration, register the body ego experience of gratification. The object impression, of the manner in which it is attained, is represented as the good instinctual aspect of the object. The background object of primary identification has established a foundation for the representation of instinctual gratification. The optimally gratifying aspects of empathic interactions enhance and expand this process.

2. The second is the mental impression of an optimally frustrating object. An object in the external world, in being empathic with the seeds of autonomous functioning in the infant, provides optimal restraint and frustration so as to evoke the exercise of those functions. It is this quality in an interaction that is represented as the optimally frustrating good object.

3. The third is the mental impression that has formed the background object of primary identification. This is represented as a transitional object and serves as the nidus for consolidating a whole good object. Empathic contact stimulates the anlage of functions within the self. The body ego experiences and object impressions that result are represented within the self, yet, the source is outside of the self. This reflects the pathway by which the background object of primary identification was originally formed and is a mirror image of a similar process occurring at the interior. (The continuum of biophysiologic demand has a dimension that is outside of the self.)

The Representations of the Bad Object

Perceptual contact with biophysiologic demands at the interior has a dimension that is potentially traumatic. It leaves a mental impression with the independent qualities of an object, which serves as the nidus for consolidating the various representations of a bad object into a whole. There are three facets:
1. One facet is represented as the bad instinctual object. This is the impression of that aspect of the continuum of instinctual demand possessing the independent qualities of an object and is overstimulating in nature. It functions as the portal of entry for instinctual activity.
2. The second is represented as an impinging object. Unempathic responses of an external object or the impact of sensory overstimulation mobilizes reactions (fight, flight, and withdrawal) that are represented in the bad self. The object impressions of these impingements resonate with the instinctual impingements at the interior and coalesce.
The Big Black Pops in A were examples of these impinging representations of an object. The Make-A-Dos also possessed qualities of impingement but with an instinctual dimension. In addition, there was a line of continuity from pleasurable, to anxiety arousing, to being portrayed as a bad instinctual object. The Big Black Pops were prohibitive in nature and patterned after interactions with an object in the external world.
3. The third is represented as a depriving object. These are the object impressions of the inevitable experiences of sensory deprivation.

The Interrelationship of the Self- and Object Representational Systems

As perceptual maturation advances, the distant perceptual functions of hearing and sight become more functional. They exert an organizational influence, and their activity is more capable of representation. The empathic activity of external objects evoke and resonate with the seeds of autonomous functions and amplify their use. These ego functions become more available to engage in the processes that further the representation of the demands of biophysiology and expand the body ego experience of instinctual gratification. The boundaries of the self are expanded as the part object impressions consolidate into the representation of a whole good and bad object. This system of object representations is forming as a structured manifestation of the effects of interactions and of the manner in which perceptual activity is elicited.

The impingements and deprivations created by objects in the external world are represented as the impinging and depriving facets of the bad object and coalesce with the instinctual impingements represented as the bad instinctual object (the nidus for organizing a whole bad object). The empathic activities of objects in the external world are represented as the optimally gratifying and optimally frustrating facets of the good object and coalesce with the representation of a transitional object (the nidus for organizing a whole good object). The representations of a good object consolidate at the periphery, separate from the representations of a bad object that consolidates at the interior. A line of continuity of experience is maintained as the restraining influence of optimal frustration, represented in the good object, gradually blends through prohibitions into the impingements represented in the bad object.

Interactions with an external object are the source of continuing body ego experiences of containment, gratification, and amplification of the anlagen of autonomous ego functions. These body ego experiences and object impressions are represented as facets of the good self and good object. These interactions are also the source of impingements and deprivations, which are represented as the varied facets of the bad self and bad object. When the good qualities of experience are sufficient and the bad qualities are not inordinate, they facilitate the processes of advancing differentiation.

Empathic interactions occur at the periphery, but the body ego experiences are drawn to the interior where the part good self-representations are coalescing. Instinctual demand requiring defense transpires at the interior, but the body ego experiences are drawn to the periphery where the part bad self-representations are coalescing. This translocation of perception is the basis for the splitting mechanisms that express the defensive activity of the primitively organized ego. The advancing experience of phase-specific instinctual gratification enhances the binding funciton of libidinal activity and forms a more solidly consolidated representation of the good self. When there is sufficient structuralization of unified representations of a good self at the interior to offer stability, the continuing process of consolidation moves closer to the periphery. In conjunction with the increasing maturation of the perceptual processes and the further consolidation of good object impressions, it gradually becomes possible to perceive the object as the source of empathic responsiveness. This development strengthens the structured good self-representations and fosters their movement to the periphery. The resulting inner stability makes it possible for the whole bad self-representations to recede to the interior. The structuralized remnants of the reactions to impingement remain at the periphery to serve a defensive and differentiating function, and the splits in the ego are healed.

The good and bad representations of the object coalesce, maintaining a connection through a continuity of prohibitive experience (represented as optimal frustration in the good object and shading into impingements, represented in the bad object). The budding capacity to recognize a good object's influence, which is evolving at the periphery, can only be realized by extending the activity of perception around the structuralized remnants of reactions to impingement. This perceptual act expands the boundaries of the self and initiates the function of self-observation. When the experience is represented and structuralized, it forms the eye of consciousness. The recognition of these representations of a good object strengthens their consolidation, furthers the emergence from the lack of differentiation associated with a psychological symbiosis, and prepares the groundwork for the separation–individuation process. In the early stages, the recognition is only weakly maintained and is alternatingly established and lost. One result of this development is the expansion of the boundaries of the self and the emergence of the function of self-observation.

The advances in maturation of the autonomous ego functions, operating in concert with an increasingly defined system of self- and object representations, facilitates the inclusion of expanding dimensions of biophysiologic demand. There is more mental structure available for representation, for stability and regulation, and for advancing differentiation. The complexities of psychosexual development are manifested with the changing instinctual body ego experiences represented as the component instincts. The evolution and elaboration of a self- and object representational system enable greater quantities of instinctual activity to gain access to integration. The perceptual boundaries of the self expand, and there is a state of readiness for the formation of new mental structures that unite and differentiate the self- and object systems of representation. The prolonged dependence of the infant is related to the need for external objects to participate in interactions that provide the functions that are undeveloped. These interactions create body ego experiences, which are represented and enable the building of mental structures that establish inner regulation.

Innate deficiencies in the perceptual apparatus can have profound effects. Deficiencies in those perceptual processes, necessary for representation and/or organization, result in defects in the self-representations. This will be manifested in a lack of perceptual stability or in an unevenness in establishing the function of consensual validation so necessary for processes of integration and differentiation. Inherent deficiencies can occur at the borderland of biology and psychology. Weak or defective primal repression creates a relative intensification of biologic demand. The potential for trauma increases; there is an overdevelopment of bad self- and bad object representations and a poorly stabilized good self-representation. An innate absence or deficiency in perceptual registration at the interior will foster the overdevelopment of good self- and good object representations. This can make differentiation and the process of separation–individuation relatively ineffective. The motivating force for continuing development will be minimal, fusion and merger body ego experiences will predominate, and a more fixed symbiotic configuration will influence all advances in development.

The Process of Separation–Individuation

The initial perception of the object as separate from the self is tenuous, unstable, and difficult to sustain. This perception is stabilized by the recognition of the continuity of prohibitive experience, represented as optimal frustration in the good object and shading into the impingements represented in the bad object. This stabilized perception of the separateness of the self and object (in both the internal and external world) is an important condition for these systems to be linked through the formation of new structures. There are tenuous connections that have already been established through the lines of continuity of instinctual and prohibitive experience. The line of continuity of instinctual experience, in the self-representational system, extends tenuously to the instinctual representation of the bad object. The line of continuity of prohibitive experience, in the object representational system, extends tenuously to the reactions to impingement represented in the bad self.

The consolidation and structuralization of the representations of good self-experience have evolved during the symbiotic period, in a state of lack of differentiation. Thus the initial tenuous recognition of the good object as separate is very unstable and necessitates the active utilization of all available perceptual functions. The activity of these autonomous functions are represented to form an eye of consciousness, which is very difficult to sustain. The temporary loss of this perceptual focus, with fatigue or stress, is associated with anxiety. However, once the pathway has formed, the capacity to reestablish this developmental progression is readily available.

The optimally frustrating activities of an external object are represented as a facet of the good object because they evoke and amplify the body ego experiences of autonomous functioning that are represented in the good self. The aspect of restraint gradually shades into the impingements represented in the bad object. It is this perception of the good object's bad qualities that stabilizes the experience of self-differentiation. The evolving eye of consciousness is enhanced, and with it the function of self-observation.

The developing infant now has a differentiating influence within the personality, founded upon a relatively stabilized connection of the self- and object systems of representation. A functional eye of consciousness further enhances the experience of differentiation and establishes the necessary conditions for the process of separation–individuation to take place. In addition, the expanded boundaries of the self have created a sector of transitional space. This is the psychological space created by extending perceptual activity to move around the structured remnants of reactions to impingement, to locate the representation of a whole good object. It is at this point in development that the infant utilizes a transitional object as a stimulus to evoke the representations of a good object. The original body ego experience of contact with the maternal intrauterine environment has been represented as the background object of primary identification in the good self. In this very primitive state of perception, there is a trace of an object impression that will evolve as the nidus around which the mental impressions of a good object organize. The maternal environment is the first transitional object, and it is registered to provide the necessary background for the formation of an object representational system. A transitional object, in eliciting the memory traces of a good object's influence, diminishes the stress on the newly established self-expansion. When there is sufficient stability for the connection between the self- and object systems of representation to be sustained, two poles of mental activity result. One is along the pathway of the self-representations and facilitates introjective processes. The other is along the pathway of the object representations and facilitates projective processes.

The "Bipolar" Self: The Introjective and Projective Arms of Perception

The search for, and location of, the representation of a good object has enabled a perceptual attunement to the internal world that is reflected in the development of the eye of consciousness. The structured remnants of reactions to impingement, at the periphery, have served a defensive function and obscure the perception of a good object. The effect is to enhance the growing experience of differentiation. It also creates the necessity for a perceptual movement around these reactions to impingement, in order to identify the good object in the external world and the representations of a good object in the internal world. Initially, this expanded self-boundary is tenuous and easily lost. Body ego experiences with a good object in a less differentiated state exert a strong regressive pull. These are the symbiotic fusion and merger experiences that were essential in consolidating the representations of a whole good self. Fluctuations of expansion and retraction continue until this advancing perceptual boundary becomes stabilized. The establishment of a perceptual connection to the representation of a good object (around the reactions to impingement) forms the eye of consciousness, transitional space, and an introjective and projective arm of perception. The recognition of the good object's bad qualities stabilizes this perceptual and structural position. A clearly defined separate relationship between the self- and object representational systems has evolved. This is a relationship of body ego experience to the object impressions that created them; it stabilizes the perceptions of the inner world and forms a skeletal foundation for the expression of an individual's character.

A dual perceptual function becomes manifested and operational at the point of contact with the external world. This is the perception of the external world and the function of self-observation in the inner world. The self has now evolved into a bipolar configuration. *Bipolar* refers to the development of an object representational system at one pole and a self-representational system at the other. The formation of the eye of consciousness has extended the boundaries of the self to link one pole to the other. The perceptual movement, around the structured remnants of reactions to impingement, has formed an introjective arm of perception. This provides the perceptual pathway for introjective mechanisms to operate. The perception of a whole good object representation, which is stabilized by a recognition of its bad qualities, has formed a projective arm of perception. This provides the perceptual pathway for projective mehcanisms to operate. Mirroring activities will be introjected and be evocative to the self-representational system. Idealizing processes will be elaborated on the projective arm of perception.

The emergence of a "bipolar" self can only occur with the gradual diminution of splitting mechanisms as the predominant defense of the ego. The earlier translocations of perception are rectified as the represented good self rises to the periphery and the bad self recedes into the interior. Mental impressions of good self-experience (optimal gratification, optimal frustration, and a transition object) have been represented and coalesce at the periphery. Mental impressions of bad self-experience (instinctual from contact with the traumatic dimension of the self with object qualities, impinging from contact with unempathic external objects and depriving from the inevitable sensory deprivations) have been represented and coalesce at the interior. Thus the representations of good experience are organizing at the point of perceptual contact with the external world and bad experiences at the point of perceptual contact with biophysiologic demands and bodily processes.

The structured remnants of reactions to impingement remain at the periphery where they serve a protective, differentiating function and foster a perceptual orientation to the external world. The structured representations of a good self remain at the interior where they serve a stabilizing function and buffer the impact of biophysiologic demand. When the boundaries of the self expand, the outer border of the eye of consciousness and the introjective and projective arms of perception are perceptually attuned to the external world, from the influence of the reactions to impingement. The inner border of th eye of consciousness and the introjective and projective arms of perception are perceptually attuned to the inner world, from the influence of the search for a represented good object.

In summary, the whole good object has three represented facets: optimal gratification, optimal frustration, and the transitional object. The representation of the transitional object serves as a nidus around which the other aspects of goodness consolidate into a whole. The whole bad object has three represented facets: instinctual, impinging, and depriving. The instinctual aspect, derived from contact with the overstimulating dimension of the self with object qualities, serves as a nidus around which the other aspects of badness consolidate into a whole. The object representational system evolves as a consequence of interactions with the external world and with the traumatic dimensions of instinctual demand in the internal world. The perception of the object representational system, with its good and bad qualities, fosters differentiation. Fusion and merger body ego experiences cannot take place as long as this percepton is maintained. The boundaries of the self expand when perceptual activity is directed to a search for the representation of a good object. The representations of autonomous functioning are extended into an introjective arm of perception. This is the pathway of perceptual movement around the structured remnants of reactions to impingement. The location of the representation of a good object, associated with the recognition of its bad qualities, stabilizes that perception and forms a projective arm of perception. These two arms of perception function as extensions of the two poles of the self, the introjective arm as an extension of the self-representations and the projective arm as an extension of the object representations.

Discussion

In both patients, when the therapeutic interaction was unconsciously empathic and experienced as containing, a clearer picture of the composition of the self- and object representational systems became apparent. In *A*, the Make-A-Dos were instinctual in nature. The anal qualities of mastery, control, and mischievousness were a reflection of their representation as a part of the good self. The manner in which these objects occupied his mind was a manifestation of the inner fragmentation that was present. The name of these objects also revealed their anal characteristics. A line of continuity of instinctual experience was evident in their representation, as a part of the bad self, with dangerous qualities requiring defense. As instinctual intensity increased, the line of continuity was extended to their representation with the ominous instinctual qualities of a bad object.

The representations of a whole good self were only available in the presence of the containing function of the background object of primary identification. The instinctual facet was expressed in the joyful activities of the Make-A-Dos. The utilization of autonomous ego functions was only intermittently available. The ability to maintain a consolidated whole good self was tenuous and dependent upon the unconsciously empathic qualities of the therapeutic interaction. The representations of a bad self were most clearly portrayed by the figure of Pa-Ba, in which the aspects of deprivation and reactions to impingement predominated. These were split off from the dangerous, instinctual Make-A-Dos, which had a fragmenting effect. Pa-Ba was a deprived, impinged-upon, impaired, maimed, and helpless infant. This representation of a bad self highlighted its oral characteristics and reflected the severe damage incurred very early in development.

The figures of The Big Pain and Big Black Pops were manifestations of the fragmented, poorly consolidated aspects of the bad object. The ominous object qualities of the Make-A-Dos reflected the disruptive effects of intensified instinctual demand. The Big Pain represented an object that elicited painful experiences, had only the most minimal capacity to offer optimal gratification, and was predominantly depriving in nature. This object representation expressed the influence of contact with the maternal figure in the external world. The Big Black Pops were highly threatening in nature and portrayed the manner in which prohibitions were experienced. They were patterned after the paternal figure in the external world, and the name symbolically captured the explosive effect of their prohibitive influence as well as the figure that participated in their formation. Good object impressions possessing attributes of optimal frustration were initially nonexistent.

The soldier was a new representation of an object, emerging during the course of the therapeutic situation. Good object qualities of optimal gratification, optimal frustration, and of a transitional object were only consolidated in this figure. All other representations of an object were of badness and were poorly consolidated.

In *C*, the representations of the self and object and of their lines of continuity of instinctual and prohibitive experience were more apparent. This was a function of the higher level of psychic organization that had been a part of his development. The instinctual aspect of the good self was represented in the thoughts of *Playboy* and the associated sexual excitement. The line of continuity of instinctual experience could be traced, as the bad self-representations emerged, with memories of masturbatory activities accompanied by shame and embarrassment. This progressed with building intensity to the poorly represented inner experience of danger that had the qualities of a bad instinctual object. The autonomous ego functions, represented in the good self, were expressed in the thoughts of activities in which he was effective in the use of his skills. Sensory deprivation, represented in the bad self, was portrayed in his recollections of unrealized potentials. The remembrance of the country, associated with a feeling of containment, manifested the qualities of the background object of primary identification. The reactions to impingement, represented in the bad self, were pictured in the memories of rage and retreat in response to intimidating figures. These are reminiscent of the fight, flight, and withdrawal responses that characterize reactions to impingement.

The representations of the object's good and bad qualities and the line of continuity of prohibitive experience were also displayed. The representations of the father as a restraining, frustrating figure quickly shifted into impinging and attacking qualities. The composition of this figure was a manifestation of the paucity of representations of optimal frustration and of the ready and rapid transition to prohibitions and impingement. The optimally gratifying representations of a good object were portrayed in the empathic activities of the mothering figure. This representation readily shifted into a figure that was easily controlled and possessed the instinctual qualities of a bad object.

The therapist was able to maintain a consistent nonimpinging, empathically responsive interaction with C. Although C exerted intense interactional pressure upon the therapist to elicit responses that would reinforce his defensive postures, the interaction was unconsciously perceived as containing. This was expressed in his feeling of relief, his deprecatory teasing, and in his gradually revealing the extent of his inner disturbance. The qualities of containment in the interaction made it possible for pathological distortions to become accessible for alteration, integration, and change.

The concept of the self with object qualities was helpful in explaining the variable characteristics of the Make-A-Dos. They were given one name, though they shifted from being pleasurable and not requiring defense, to being overstimulating and requiring defense, to being ominous and assuming the proportions of an independent, instinctually threatening object. This would indicate that they emanated from one source. They seemed to represent the effects of biophysiologic demands and gave some definition to the original body ego experience by which a stimulus outside of the self could be included within the self.

The concept of the object with self-qualities seemed to offer a construct to explain the manner in which new representational structures are formed. The soldier reflected the effects of the therapeutic interaction and possessed attributes consonant with the qualities of goodness. When the therapist's unconsciously empathic responsiveness was consistent and uninterrupted, *A* seemed to experience a lack of differentiation. He molded to the body of the therapist, gave directions as to how to buffer the impact of stimuli, and appeared to be immersed in an internal state of lack of differentiation. During this period, a stimulus outside of the self (the interaction with the therapist) was included within the self (a firmer representation of a good self and the new representation of the soldier). The effect was to amplify and expand upon the containing function of the background object of primary identification. *A*'s ability to maintain a consolidated whole good self-representation was tenuous and dependent upon the unconsciously empathic qualities of the therapeutic interaction.

C experienced the fragmenting panic of his separation anxiety and invoked within himself the listening, integrating (containing and metabolizing) attitude of the therapist. The associative chain of thoughts and imagery reflected the varying representations of the self and object and their lines of continuity. The fragmented part self- and part object representations were consolidating into a whole under the organizing influence of the background object of primary identification. The differing aspects of body ego experiences, which are represented to comprise a whole, are most in evidence when they are in a state of fragmentation (as in *A*), or in the process or organization (as in *C*).

CHAPTER 3

Libido as Object Seeking and the Mechanism of Splitting

An Integration of Libidinal and Object Relations Theory

Introduction

When I was exposed to psychoanalytic theory, those concepts that made a connection to my experiences in the past and present were internalized. The theory of libido and psychosexual development was amply verified on innumerable occasions and became integrated into my manner of listening and responding to the inner experiences of others. My awareness of the significance of the therapeutic interaction increased, and one aspect of libidinal theory kept returning to me as difficult to grasp. The theory portrayed instinctual activity as primarily discharge seeking, yet the simple act of libidinal discharge did not effect therapeutic change. Change was associated with the ascendency of healthy adaptive processes and seemed to occur in response to the effects of an interaction. In addition, as far as I could determine, libidinal activity was manifested only in contact with an object and the representations of an object. Many others had made similar observations. Some had even suggested that libidinal theory be discarded altogether. I was intrigued by Fairbairn's writing but troubled by his inability to integrate libido as object seeking and still maintain the usefulness of libidinal theory in the exploration of instinctual experience. It had been easy to accept the totality of libidinal theory because it did explain so much. However, the theory had not been fully reconsidered after the development of the structural theory, and it seemed to me that an integration of libidinal and object relations theory was demonstrable. I thought it would be important to establish the relationship of libidinal activity to structure formation and formulate a developmental metapsychological construct that could define the original object of libidinal activity.

In working with more primitively organized patients, I came in contact with the effects of splitting mechanisms upon the internal world of mental representations. The splitting mechanism operated to maintain an adaptive split of the good and bad qualities of self-experience, which appeared to facilitate a consolidation of the part self-representations into a whole. This observation required an explanation. If libidinal activity only sought discharge, it would not be necessary to divide perceptual experience into separate areas of representation. Furthermore, it required the mental impression of an object for this mechanism to be operative. In more organized personalities, where continuity of experience was established and repression proper was the primary defense, the idea of libido as discharge seeking was consonant with clinical observations. My impression was that one significant difference between primitively organized patients and those with higher levels of organization was a result of the degree to which early splits in the ego had been healed. Thus it would also be important to delineate the manner in which this developmental task was negotiated.

Patients, in whom the splitting mechanism was continually active, initially responded to contact with the stimuli of the external world with the qualities of bad self-experience. These same patients, when a therapeutic interaction was empathically responsive to unconscious communications, revealed the presence of qualities of good self-experience. These qualities of goodness seemed to have been represented and consolidated at the interior and were tenuous, vulnerable, and easily disrupted. When they were impinged upon, deprived, or overstimulated, profound states of fragmentation were precipitated.

Patients, who were more organized, appeared to react with qualities of good self-experience to the stimuli of the external world. Qualities of bad self-experience would emerge in response to empathic unconscious communications. These bad qualities of self-experience appeared to have been represented and consolidated at the interior. These same patients gave evidence of having structured the representations of good self-experience so that their influence was present throughout the personality. It is a frequent observation with infants that irritability and reactions to impingement are immediately evident in response to unfamiliar or unempathic stimuli. These reactions imply that qualities of bad self-experience are represented and organize at the point of contact with the external world. The same infant responds to an empathic interaction with the emergence of qualities of good self-experience. A metapsychology, that includes the concept of libido as object seeking, emphasizes the primacy of interractions. I will attempt to describe the source of the earliest representations that serve as an object for libido and the manner in which the varying aspects of libidinal activity are represented. I will also indicate the significance of the mechanism of splitting and the necessity of this mechanism for furthering developmental progression.

Clinical Material

After a time, the quality of *A*'s being held began to change. *A* was quiet, contained, and molded himself to the body of the therapist with little animation, irritability, or expression of any intensity. *A* developed a pattern of entering the room and passively establishing physical contact with the therapist. He brought in the injured and erect soldiers once again. He played with them in a listless manner and behaviorally indicated the interchangeability of the two soldiers. The therapist stated that being held and contained was comforting, but *A* also lost much in his ability to talk about his disturbing inner experiences. It looked to the therapist as if *A* needed him to be like the soldier, who knew when it was time to be firm. It was time for the injured soldier to use his strengths and to not be cared for in the old way. Initially, there seemed to be no response to the therapist's words and shift in attitude. *A* remained listlessly in the therapist's lap. Suddenly, *A* arose, walked to the other side of the room, and spoke directly to the therapist. In reference to an upcoming interruption, necessitated by the therapist's vacation, A asked, "Dr. go way?" His uncertain, questioning tone expressed his anxiety concerning the distance he experienced in what had just transpired.

D was a 17-year-old girl who entered therapy following an active suicidal attempt. She was terrified over her loss of control and of her periodic experiences of inner fragmentation. D entered the following session very agitated and irritable. She felt lost and confused and began to viciously attack the therapist for being silent and unaffected by her pain and suffering. She experienced the therapist as depriving and withholding, his silence as attacking, judgmental, and critical. As she spoke, her rage mounted. The intensity was such that she appeared on the threshold of physically attacking the therapist. The therapist stated that although she appeared and sounded enraged, he could not help but feel that she was crying out to be held and contained. D immediately burst into tears. She noticed, as the therapist's words were spoken, that the sound of his words resonated with an inner longing to be soothed and comforted. She felt frightened as she talked. She felt that she had to hold these feelings deep inside; to express them carried with it a fear of inner fragmentation.

The Nature of Perceptual Activity in the Nuclear State

The perceptual processes register impressions of stimuli, which are the source of all mental experience. The nuclear self has been defined and outlined by the functioning of these perceptual processes. This concept implies that there is an element of autonomy present from the outset; that is, there is a self with boundaries. Initially, these boundaries are vague (poorly differentiated), reactive, and based upon the experiences of a body ego. The perceptual processes also register the impressions of the world of stimuli that are independent of this nuclear self. The body ego experiences and object impressions that create them are then mentally represented. The process of representation transpires within boundaries determined by the activity of perception. As the state of perception changes, the boundaries of the self change. It is thereby important to conceptualize the nature of perceptual activity in the nuclear state and to trace the evolution of perceptual activity through the advancing stages of development.

With the dawning of perception, a primordial nuclear self emerges. The perceptual modalities that are most intimately linked to bodily functions have the greatest impact and exert the strongest influence upon the registration of body ego experiences. These near receptors—of touch, temperature, taste—are most instrumental in establishing the boundaries of a nuclear self. The distant receptors—of hearing and sight—have a lesser impact and a minimal influence upon the initial boundaries that are formed. The perceptual processes have the effect of awakening and amplifying the representational and organizing functions of the primitive (primary body) ego. The near receptors are more powerful in evoking representational functions and have little effect upon the ego's organizing capacities. The distant receptors exert only a minimal effect on the representational functions but have the potential to strongly activate organizational functions.

The varied aspects of body ego experience consolidate into the representation of a whole good and bad self, as the perceptual modalities are integrated into a functional unity. The representational capacities of the ego that have been associated with the near receptors become available to the distant receptors, and the organizing capacities of the ego that have been associated with the distant receptors become available to the near receptors. Consensual validation is then functional within the personality. The first manifestation of the effective establishment of consensual validation is the recognition of the external object and its representation as separate.

The world of biophysiology exerts a constant impact upon the perceptual processes. However, not all dimensions of this biophysiologic demand are capable of being perceived. The demands of biophysiology are on a continuum that is continuously present within the organism. The state of integration of the perceptual processes and the available mental impressions will determine how this continuum of demands is perceived and represented. I have named, as mentioned previously, the continuum of biophysiologic demand as "the self with object qualities." I have done so to incorporate the totality of the continuum and to emphasize that there is an aspect that is independent of perception, and thus functionally, has the effects of an object. There is a segment that is represented with no need for defense, a segment that is over-stimulating and represented requiring defense, a segment that has the effect of an impinging object, and a segment that is beyond the boundaries of the self and not represented. The demands of biophysiology are thus on a continuum with what is inside of the self, which ranges to what is within the organism but outside of the self.

Deprivations refer to sensory deprivations. They exist to some extent in all individuals because it is impossible to maintain contact with sensory modalities at all times. The very presence of a focus of perceptual attention in one realm obviates against its presence in another. In addition, the external world may have limitations in providing empathically attuned sensory experience. When such deprivations are excessive, it will be reflected in the body ego experience of weakness or atrophy in the autonomous ego functions. Frustration is related to instinctual activity and indicates the absence of gratification. Impingements are the result of stimuli that mobilize a defensive response, are too intense, or are traumatic. When a given stimulus is registered, with insufficient representational structure to allow the delay necessary to institute defense, it is traumatic. Any impingement has a defensive and potentially traumatic aspect. Impingements and the reactions to them are essential for faciliating the processes of defense and differentiation.

The Original Object for Libidinal Representation

Instinct has been defined as the manner in which the demands of biophysiology are represented in the psyche. In the original formulation, prior to the structural hypotheses, instinct was presented as discharge seeking. In developing a concept of libido as object seeking, it is essential to offer a metapsychological definition of the original object that is available for libidinal representation. The implications of this alteration in theory are vast. It eliminates the idea of a primary narcissistic state and adds a foundation for determining the role of interactions with an external object for the development of the self. It also implies that psychic structuralization begins *in utero*.

The dawning of the activity of perceptual processes registers a body ego experience of the physiological, metabolic, buffering interactions with the maternal uterine environment. With the impact of this stimulus, the representational functions of the primitive ego are activated, and a primordial nuclear self is born. The act of perception initiates the formation of a boundary that, *in utero,* is poorly differentiated. The body ego experience of these metabolizing, containing, buffering functions of the physiological surrounding of the mother is represented as the background object of primary identification. It is this representation that is available as a foundation for stimuli outside of the self to be introjected and to be included through representation within the self. An element of biophysiological demand is now capable of representation. Libidinal demand treats this representation as an object, and, in not requiring defense, it is registered as the initial part good self-representation of phase-specific instinctual gratification. This part good self-representation has required an interaction with an object (the intrauterine environment) in order to evolve. Thus the state of primary narcissism would only refer to that period of development prior to the functioning of perceptual processes.

The Developmental Significance of Splitting

Throughout the course of development, increasing quantities of instinctual demand are included, through representation, within the self. The nature of instinctual representation changes, in conjunction with the effects of maturation, the progression in perceptual integration, and the changing conditions of instinctual gratification. The advancing stages of instinctual representation emerge as an evolution of the component instincts and their eventual consolidation into a genital drive. There is always an aspect of biophysiological demand that does not require defense, an aspect that requires defense, and an aspect with a perceptual impact having the qualities of an overstimulating object. I have called this continuum as mentioned previously, "the self with object qualities," and it is represented as the instinctual facet of the good self, the bad self, and the bad object. There is also a dimension that is incapable of representation.

Interactions with external objects present stimuli and elicit responses that are also on a continuum. Empathic interactions are optimally gratifying and optimally frustrating and evoke the representation of the background object of primary identification. During the symbiotic period, these empathic activities are perceived in a state of lack of differentiation and have self-qualities. The same external object, in providing the restraints of optimal frustration, invariably introduces elements of impingement. In addition, the impossibility of amplifying all sensory modalities simultaneously carries with it some inevitable degree of sensory deprivation. The continuum is registered with the mental impressions of an object that will be represented as a facet of the good object (optimal gratification and optimal frustration), the bad object (impinging and depriving), and expand a facet of the good self (the background object and the experience of instinctual gratification). I have called this continuum, as mentioned previously "the object with self-qualities." The variable body ego experiences and object impressions that result from a single source of stimulation, one in the external world and one in the internal world, are initially represented as separated from each other. A background for the mechanism of splitting is thus accessible to the early, primitive ego.

Good self-experience is sufficiently variable to be registered separately and gradually consolidates into the representation of a whole good self. There are three facets: the background object of primary identification, the phase-specific instinctual gratifications, and the activity of autonomous ego functions. Each represented aspect serves a specific function. The autonomous ego functions define the boundaries of the self; the background object of primary identification provides the foundation for expanding representational structures; and the phase-specific instinctual gratifications assert the binding function of libidinal activity. Maturation of the perceptual processes is interrelated with the evolving systems of mental representation, and the boundaries of the self are expanded.

A whole good self-representation consolidates at the interior, though the interaction that enables it is occurring at the periphery. The representations of good self-experience coalesce at the site at which the background object of primary identification is represented. This is the area of peceptual contact with the demands of biophysiology, and libidinal activity exerts its demand for representation at this locale. The aspect of biophysiologic demand that is overstimulating also exerts its effects at the interior. This dimension of instinctual activity has an impinging quality.

A whole bad self-representation consolidates at the periphery, though its instinctual facet has been registered at the interior. The representations of bad self-experience coalesce at this site to serve a protective and differentiating function. The impingements of the external world have a powerful impact, which stimulates the reactions of fight, flight, and withdrawal that are represented as a facet of the bad self. They combine with the interior impingements of instinctual overstimulation and the experiences of sensory deprivation to organize at this area of perceptual contact with the external world. This process, which involves a translocation of perception. is the mechanism of splitting. A stimulus at the periphery is represented at the interior, and a stimulus at the interior is represented at the periphery.

When the representations of good self-experience are sufficiently consolidated at the interior, the disruptive effects of biophysiologic demand are buffered. The impact of biophysiologic demand can then operate as a stimulus for further differentiation, and the organizing representations of a good self can rise to the surface. A foundation of stability is present within the personality that, in conjunction with the increasing capacity for self-differentiation, allows empathic interactions to be registered and represented where they occur. Concurrently, the representations of a bad self recede into the interior where the overstimulating dimension of instinctual demand continues to exert its effects. The structured remnants of reactions to impingement remain at the periphery maintaining a differentiating influence, and the structured remnants of a good self remain at the interior maintaining a stabilizing influence. The translocations of perception are then no longer necessary to facilitate ongoing expansion in the representations of self-experience.

The evolving sequence in organizing the representations of self-experience, and their object-impression counterparts, reflects the progression in perceptual maturation and establishment of consensual validation. The varied representations of good self-experience consolidate into a whole, abetted by the mechanism of splitting. The representations of bad self-experience, which have been coalescing, then organize into an entity. At this point, the object impressions of good qualities coalesce at the periphery and of bad qualities at the interior. The mental impression of a transitional object serves as a nidus around which the impressions of optimal gratification and optimal frustration coalesce, to ultimately be represented as a whole good object. The mental impression of instinctual demand that impacts upon the perceptual processes with the independent qualities of an object serves as a nidus around which the impressions of impingement and deprivation coalesce, to ultimately be represented as a whole bad object.

The Foundation for Processes of Internalization and the Relationship to Splitting

The nature of self-experience changes as progressions in development are manifested. Self-experience *in utero*, or at birth, differs markedly from the experience of the self at various stages throughout life. The connections from the earliest to the more advanced forms of self-experience can be made through an understanding of a particular developmental line. For example, the core of self-experience that is objectless and is present in the infant *in utero* ultimately becomes the core of separateness upon which identity is built.

With the dawning of perception, core body ego experiences are registered reflecting a connection to stimuli that are simultaneously outside of, and a part of, the self. That connection is occurring at two locales. One is at the periphery, with the containing, physiological buffering, and metabolizing functions of the maternal environment. This connection is so attuned to, and responsive to, elements within the self that it is experienced as undifferentiated from the self. The reactive object impression is of a stimulus outside of the self that is buffering, containing, metabolizing, and digesting. The body ego experience is represented as the background object of primary identification, which evolves as the background for the expression of all mental events. (The experience is not always one of containment. Deficiencies in the infant and/or the mother may be disruptive.) The representations of this body ego experience are at the foundation of the psychological symbiosis of postuterine life. The background object of primary identification provides an introjective pathway for the infant to experience empathic contact with the external world, inside of the self.

The second locale is at the interior, where there is perceptual contact with the continuum of biophysiological demand. A segment is registered, represented, and included within the self without defense; an element is impinging and necessitates defense; there is an aspect that is traumatic with the qualities of an independent, overstimulating object and a dimension that is unrepresentable, yet within the organism. This continuum of biophysiological demand has such a variable impact that it is represented differently, though it emanates from a single source of stimulation. The segment included within the self without defense is represented as the instinctual aspect of the good self. The element that is impinging and necessitates defense is represented as the instinctual aspect of the bad self. The aspect that is traumatic elicits a perceptual impression that is functionally experienced as an overstimulating object and is represented as the instinctual aspect of the bad object. This facet of the internal world is on a continuum with the dimension that is not representable. It is the portal of entry, into the self, of a source of stimulation that is the most threatening and defended against.

The empathic activities of an external object are also on a continuum. One aspect is optimally gratifying, which evokes the body ego experience represented as phase-specific instinctual gratification. However, optimal gratification can only take place when coexistent with optimal frustration. The optimally frustrating aspect requires a sensitive awareness of the budding autonomous functions in the infant and amplifies the body ego experience of their use. Restraint embodies some degree of prohibition, and there is also an aspect that is impinging and nonempathic. In addition, the same external object cannot provide sensory stimulation in all spheres at all times and hence is depriving. When this continuum of good and bad qualities is in proportion, the effect is to expand the representations of good self-experience necessary for growth and provide the representations of bad self-experience that facilitates defense and differentiation. The body ego experiences of empathic interactions are taking place at the periphery and are represented at the interior (consolidating around the background object of primary identification). The body ego experience of biophysiological overstimulation, which is taking place at the interior, is represented at the periphery (consolidating around the reactions to impingement from the impact of birth). This translocation of perception is the mechanism of splitting. It is the primary defensive activity available in this primitive level of organization. The healing of the splits is accomplished when development has advanced sufficiently for the representations of an experience to occur at the site of the stimulus.

Libido as Object Seeking

Libidinal instinctual activity was originally described as discharge seeking. This hypothesis was offered prior to the structural hypothesis and not returned to for alteration. The assumption that libido is discharge seeking implies that the primary task in treatment centers upon fostering those processes that facilitate the discharge of libido. Yet it is the therapeutic interaction that is crucial in treatment, not simply the discharge of libido. Some authors have defined *libido* as object seeking (especially Fairbairn, (1954). The effort to define libido as object-seeking has often led to the elimination of, or the alteration of, the theory of libido. I feel it is important to include libidinal theory because it is so useful in understanding psychosexual experience.

The representation of the background object of primary identification reflects the body ego experience of perceptual contact with the containing and metabolizing functions of the intrauterine environment. It has emerged from contact with an object, serves as a nidus for the coalescence of good self-experience, and is the original mental impression available for representation of libidinal activity. Libido is thus established as object seeking from the beginning. This aspect of instinctual demand does not require defense and is represented as the initial experience of phase-specific instinctual gratification. The continuum of biophysiological demands elicits variable impressions that are represented as the instinctual facet of the bad self or bad object, depending upon the degree of defense required. Higher levels of intensity cannot be included within self-experience even with the aid of defense and are registered with the qualities of an overstimulating instinctual object.

The experience of ongoing contact with an empathically responsive external object is evocative to the representation of the background object, amplifies its presence, establishes the conditions for a psychological symbiosis, and expands the representations of good self-experience. These external interactions are also on a continuum (the object with self-qualities) that embodies optimally gratifying, optimally frustrating, prohibiting, impinging, and depriving qualities. The balance in representation of good and bad self-experiences, in conjunction with their object-impression counterparts, provides the wherewithal to facilitate growth and differentiation.

The binding function of libido is expressed in attaching to the representation of an object and in consolidating the part self-representations into a whole. When there are sufficient quantities of good self-experience structuralized at the interior, the resulting stability enables the perceptual boundaries of the self to expand. The object impressions that have been coalescing are then organized and become more available for libidinal representation.

The maturation and activity of the perceptual processes is intimately interrelated with the organization of the self-and object representations. When perceptual processes function in isolation (as occurs in extreme pathology), the end products of their activity are concrete and fragmented. The greater the dimension of the continuum of biophysiologic demand that can be represented and integrated within the self, the more complete is the realization of potentials, and the more there is meaning to human experience.

Discussion

It is extremely difficult to determine the meaning of a given communication with a child such as *A*. So much is dependent upon the therapist's interactive responses, sensitivities, and imagination. However, when such an individual becomes verbally communicative, that very act of communication is indicative of the

utilization of autonomous ego functions, which are otherwise unavailable. Further, when the communication is specifically directed
to the therapist, it highlights the child's ability, at the moment,
to maintain a representational connection to an object. That connection reflects the effect of the relationship upon him. The actual
question, "Doctor, go way?", though subject to a variety of interpretations as to its meaning, required that the represented qualities of good self-experience be consolidated. The stimulus was a
shift in the therapist's attitude. The therapist indicated an unwill-
ingness to comfort A at the expense of his continuing growth and
development. The therapist felt, as he held A and witnessed the
change in A's behavior, that he did not want A to be helpless and
undifferentiated. For the therapist, A's internal state was of a helpless, undifferentiated crippled infant. The therapist recalled the
play with the two soldiers. When A was interchanging the positions of the injured and upright soldier, it appeared to the therapist that he was reflecting in his behavior the internal state of lack
of differentiation. The qualities of badness were dominating his inner experience and embodied his earlier description of Pa-ba, the
helpless injured infant. These qualities of badness appeared to be
at the periphery, at the point of contact with the stimuli of the external environment. The shift in the therapist's attitude and resulting statement that it was time for A to use his strengths came from
the therapist's understanding that the representations of good self-
experience were now stronger, more effective, and capable of function. Furthermore, the therapist felt that A was unconsciously indicating their presence. A, in reacting to the psychological distance
of the therapist's optimally frustrating attitude, responded with
his communicative question. He displayed an immediate sensitivity
to the separatness, which reminded him of the upcoming interruption. At that moment, the consolidated representations of good
self-experience emerged to be available at the periphery, and the
qualities of badness receded into the interior. The result was not
in fragmentation but in a more consolidated expression of adaptive functioning. This gave some indication that the original splits
were, at least transiently, healed. The consolidated representations
of good self-experience came into direct perceptual contact with
an empathic external object. Momentarily, there was sufficient
structuralization of these qualities of goodness so they could rise
to the surface as the representations of bad self-experience receded

into the interior. The therapist had perceived *A* as unconsciously communicating his need for an optimally frustrating response. *A* was dependent upon the therapist to provide a sensitive awareness of *A*'s ability to function, and the shift in attitude appeared to amplify those functions. It is this influence of the therapeutic interaction that gives emphasis to the concept of libido as object seeking. It is not the discharge of libido but the particular representational structures that are evoked by the interaction that is primary. The nature of libidinal activity is then determined by the mental representations that are available.

D vividly portrayed the effects of maintaining the representations of a whole bad self at the periphery. She felt deprived, withheld from, impinged upon, attacked, and consumed with rage. The therapist, sensing the underlying instability of the background object of primary identification, addressed his communication to *D*'s inner longing for comfort and containment. The intent was to provide resonance with, and amplification of, this representation of good self-experience. The therapist thought the intensity of instinctual demand was threatening fragmentation. *D*'s immediate response was to verify the presence of an inner longing for containment and to indicate that the therapist's words had an organizing and consolidating influence. The representations of a whole good self could ascend into the immediacy of her experience in adapting to the therapeutic interaction. *D* was then filled with a longing to be soothed and comforted and, at the same time, felt the stress of fragmentation anxiety. A shift had transpired. The representations of good self-experience that had been present deep in the interior moved to the periphery, and the representations of bad self-experience receded into the interior. Libidinal demands were primarily object seeking, and the phenomenum of discharge seemed to be secondary. The frustration was directed specifically to the therapist, as was the libidinal gratification associated with her longing for comfort and containment. The therapist's interpretation was enhancing to the representations of good self-experience and fostered their engagement in the interaction. The autonomous ego functions were then more accessible for integrative processes to exert their influence.

The line of continuity of instinctual experience, represented in the good and bad selves, maintains a connection even in the presence of splitting. This provides a pathway for some degree of access to good and bad qualities when they are necessary. Thus *D* was capable of utilizing some measures of autonomous functioning in the act of communicating the experiences of badness represented at the periphery. *A* had access to some qualities of badness in order to protect the fragile representations of a good self when they rose to the surface. *A* not only suffered from splits within the ego but also from splits within the self. The part self-representations were either unconsolidated or inadequately consolidated into a whole. The consequences for language formation, symbol production, and communicative expression were such that it required the unifying effect of the therapeutic interaction for these processes to become functional.

CHAPTER 4

Separation–Individuation
The Formation of New Psychic Structures

Introduction

When I first observed a child given the label of *autism*, I was struck by the strange and paradoxical sensation that I was seeing a child who at one and the same time appeared to be incredibly strong and incredibly fragile. He was strong in what looked like a resolute and determined disengagement from the external world, in spite of struggling with apparently powerful internal forces. He was fragile in seeming overwhelmed by any adaptive demand. To the observer, he appeared extremely vulnerable. I was reminded of the powerful impact that a young infant has on the surrounding environment. The presence of an infant can dominate a situation. The infant is capable of evoking strong affects in caretakers and at the same time communicates an aura of helplessness and vulnerability. As I came to know some of these children more intimately, I began to understand in a deeper way the nature and quality of their strengths and vulnerabilities. These children had relentlessly turned away from the contaminating and impinging forces of the external world and were exquisitely aware of even its most subtle expressions. They had moved deep inside of themselves to establish intense involvements with their own bodily processes. The children might appear vulnerable to the observer, but their experience was not one of vulnerability.

I had the opportunity of forming a therapeutic relationship with a small number of such children. When it was possible to establish an empathic communicative interaction, rather than being detached, the children appeared to experience the lack of differentiation associated with fusion and merger. At these moments, intense attachments to bodily processes and bodily products were relinquished. Functions, indicative of a developmental progression that previously had been unavailable, then gradually emerged. My impression was that I was a participant in the basic processes by which psychic structuring is formed. Characteristically, when such a child was emerging from this poorly differentiated state with more available function, there was an increased sense of separateness in the relationship. It was at this time that a profound sense of vulnerability and helplessness became evident. My observations were consonant with Mahler's (1958) work on symbiosis, separation–individuation, and rapprochement. During the period of lack of differentiation, body ego experiences possessing qualities of goodness (absence of defense) seemed to be consolidating. These good qualities were manifested when I was empathically responsive to nonverbal communications and appeared to ease the experience of vulnerability.

At varying times and in differing situations, I have come in contact with individuals expressing their inner sense of dread or anxiety concerning their own mortality. The quality of the anxiety associated with ideas of death seemed to echo and resonate with some unexpressed significance. The concept that the idea of death did not exist in the unconscious seemed consonant with my observations and served to deepen my curiosity as to the source of these conscious anxieties in the unconscious realm. The impression I had was not one of resonance with an unconscious fantasy but of the activity of some reactive structure. It also seemed to me that this anxiety was universal, although it differed in degrees of intensity and in the individuals' ability to maintain it within conscious experience. For some, it was an elusive inner sensation that persisted momentarily and then seemed to slip away as an inner sense of completeness took its place. For others, it was a constant inner presence that was not alleviated. The differences had a relationship to the effectiveness with which separation–individuation was negotiated. The autistic children I worked with did not possess this quality of inner experience, until separation–individuation was negotiated.

It appeared to me that a vital internal structure was formed to balance the experiences of vulnerability and helplessness that were evoked by recognizing the separateness of the self and object. This mental structure was instinctual in nature, involved a libidinal attachment to the representation of an optimally gratifying object, and functioned to unite and differentiate the self- and object systems of representation. It also appeared to me that the body ego experiences that were represented to form a self-system, and their object-impression counterparts that were represented to form an object system, could only be connected when they had been elaborated in fantasy. The fantasies functioned as a link. The conscious idea of death, and its associated anxiety, seemed to be a reflection of the tenuousness with which this structure was maintained and of the vulnerable state it was designed to balance. Death captured the essence of human vulnerability to powerful external and internal forces.

I will describe the consolidation of object impressions into a system of object representations, the relationship of the self- and object representational systems, and the manner in which they are united and differentiated. The motivations, mechanisms, and structures underlying the process of separation–individuation will be portrayed, and a definition offered for cohesiveness in the self.

Clinical Material

A continued to alternate between passively molding himself to the therapist's body and moving away physically. He appeared lost, helpless, and vulnerable as the time approached for the therapist's departure. When the therapist returned, *A* entered his first session and immediately appeared excited at seeing the therapist. He released an accumulation of fecal matter that had been retained during the entire interruption created by the therapist's absence. The therapist's immediate inner response was one of warmth, concern, and affection. He felt the wish to clean *A* much in the manner of a young infant and to reestablish the connection interfered with by the vacation. The therapist did clean *A* but held back his immediate reaction due to a defensive inner conflict. In its place, the therapist spoke of the anger he thought *A* was expressing for having been left. A's response was to become extremely withdrawn, to retreat into his previous world of posturing and gesturing, and to become uncommunicative. This continued for an extended period of time. The therapist knew something had gone wrong but only slowly realized it had been instigated by himself. The therapist's understanding of his initial inner response deepened, and he became more aware of his inner conflict. He began to speak to A. He spoke of his need to defend himself against mothering qualities evoked by A's way of returning. He told A that he had withheld this and then defensively attributed hostility to A's communication. A slowly began to talk of his feeling of abandonment by the therapist. During the therapist's absence, he had reestablished a union with the Make-A-Dos. He had been terrified that they, too, would leave him. He maintained the union by holding on to his bowel movements. The moment he saw the therapist, there was an inner feeling of letting go. His hold on the Make-A-Dos and his bowel movements was relinguished at the same time. He felt connected to the therapist and then felt attacked by the therapist's attitude and words.

E was a 6-year-old, bright, cheerful, outgoing child. He entered therapy because of concern about periodic episodes of extreme fearfulness and clinging. He stated that he had many questions inside that were too heavy for him to carry. He wanted to see someone who would be strong enough to help him lighten the load. The early months were spent with E exploring his thoughts, feelings, and fantasies. He brought them to the therapist in the form of questions. He perceived the therapist as someone who thought about his questions and returned them to E with a statement as to their meaning. E took these statements in, and they were in fact lighter; that is, they were easier to think and talk about in this new form. The questions centered around his feeling of being too close to his mother and wanting to find in himself the ability to be more separate and not need her so much. His considerable talents and skills were encroached upon by his fear of separation from his mother. He looked to male figures as a source of identification to aid him in developing a different attitude toward his mother. He wanted to maintain a feeling of closeness, without its being so debilitating. Many questions began to focus upon the conflicts engendered by the jealousies and rivalries associated with his budding genital sexuality. This was a trigger for a defensive, regressive retreat to infantile attachments. The therapist continued to be perceived as a helping figure who could digest and interpret his inner contents and aid *E* in the process of integration.

E gradually exhibited a defensive character attitude, in which he would charm and elicit laughter in the therapist to create a distraction from some disturbing inner experience. When he succeeded, his perception of the therapist was of a provocative, seductive figure who held *E* too close in the relationship. This transference fantasy distortion was based on an unconscious perception of the therapist's defensive attitude and could only be fully understood when the therapist could see his part in it. The mother became pregnant, and *E* was filled with many deep-seated questions as to the source of the pregnancy and the potential dangerous effects of the growing fetus to the mother. The birth of the new infant was a powerful stimulus for *E*. He entered the first session following the infant's return home, at first uncharacteristically silent. He made rooting mouth movements against the therapist's couch and began to talk about the effect of the infant's cries. It felt as though he heard the cries within himself. He recognized his cry to be close to his mother. He could feel the pull toward being enveloped and taken care of. These were the feelings he worked so hard to keep at a distance. He then elaborated a fantasy of tunneling into a deep pile of snow, hollowing out a space, and crawling into a fetal position. Once inside, he could not leave the space because the tunnel had become frozen over. The only avenue to freedom from that space was to burst out through the top by thrusting himself against the roof with all of his force. He immediately shifted to talking about Halloween and the costumes he wore. Last year he had been a mummy. He was all encased and hidden from the outside world. This year he planned to wear the costume of a clown. He wanted to entertain people, to make them laugh and play tricks upon them. He then wanted to tell the therapist a funny joke. He expressed concern that the therapist would not laugh and that he would feel embarrassed. The therapist responded by stating that, as *E* began to feel what it was like to be attached to someone and then break loose and be separate, as in the tunnel, his thoughts had shifted to his ways of protecting himself from that experience. He did so by wrapping himself up like a mummy or by making others laugh. Now he wanted to make the therapist laugh. The therapist thought E was concerned because he remembered how enveloped and distrustful he felt when the therapist had laughed. E became pensive and talked more about Halloween. His mother had the best things to give of anyone, but he wanted to go on his own to get good things from others. He described his initial feeling of helplessness and vulnerability in being apart from his home and his mother's goodness. He then quickly elaborated fantastic stories of his heroic ability to deal with any danger.

Preparing for Separation–Individuation: The Healing of Splits within the Ego and the Consolidation of Object Impressions

The body ego experience of perceptual contact with the intrauterine environment is represented at the interior as the background object of primary identification. It is a core of good self-experience around which the other aspects coalesce to form a unified entity. Initially, it is represented at the source of biophysiologic demand because it serves as the original object for libidinal representation and buffers the potential disruptive effects of increases in intensity. In postuterine life, the empathic responsiveness of an external object amplifies its presence to establish the conditions of lack of differentiation necessary for a psychological symbiosis. Within that symbiotic interaction, good self-experience is represented and consolidated.

The object impression of the original intrauterine contact remains at the periphery (the point of perceptual contact). It is an impression that has the qualities of a transitional object and serves as the core around which the other mental impressions of a good object's influence coalesce. The optimally gratifying, optimally frustrating activities of an external object leave their mental impressions, which build upon this focal point to ultimately consolidate into the representation of a whole good object.

The continuum of biophysiological demand has an impact on the perceptual processes of variable intensity. The dimension not requiring defense is represented as phase-specific instinctual gratification (in the good self). Increasing intensity elicits the body ego experiences of overstimulation that require defense and are represented as a facet of the bad self. These initial body ego experiences of instinctual impingements are poorly localized, due to the primitive state of perceptual organization.

The experience of birth is one of a massive impingement. The infant is suddenly confronted with profound differences in temperature, pressure, and physiologic responses. This enormous impingement elicits the body ego experiences of fight, flight, or withdrawal that are represented as a facet of the bad self at the periphery. There is a resonance with the original instinctual impingements, which are then perceptually drawn to coalesce at the site of the trauma of birth. It is this translocation of perception, within the self-system of representations, that defines the mechanism of splitting. The body ego experience of empathic perceptual contact occurring at the periphery is represented at the interior, and the body ego experience of overstimulation occurring at the interior is represented at the periphery.

The further dimension of biophysiological demand is of an intensity that is extending beyond the capacity for representation. This creates a mental impression, at the interior, possessing the qualities of an independent, overstimulating object. It is a powerful stimulus and serves as a nidus around which the other mental impressions of a bad object's influence coalesce. The unempathic, impinging, and depriving activities of an external object leave their mental impressions, which build upon this core to consolidate into the representation of a whole bad object.

When the representations of good self-experience have been of a sufficient degree, they are consolidated and structuralized at the interior. This provides a buffering presence to modulate the impact of biophysiologic demand. Their continuing process of consolidation and expansion then moves toward the periphery, the site of the ongoing stimuli of empathic interactions. The impact of biophysiologic demand which has been potentially traumatic, is more readily registered and operates as a motivating force for advancing differentiation. Concurrently, the representations of bad self-experience that have been consolidating at the periphery recede into the interior, the site of instinctual overstimulation. Their structured remnants remain at the periphery to provide a differentiating, protective influence. This development is a manifestation of the healing of the original splits within the ego and is a necessary condition for the instigation of the processes of separation and individuation. The body ego experiences, evoked by empathic contact and instinctual overstimulation, are represented at the same site as the source of the stimulus.

Separation–individuation involves the gradual perception of the good object as separate from the self. The fusion–merger experiences of the symbiotic period have facilitated the buildup of good self-representations and their object impressions and enabled the healing of splits and coalescense of object impressions into evolving entities. The representations of a whole good self have to be well established and consolidated, and the varied impressions of a good object's influence have to be sufficiently organized for the representation of a whole good object to be perceived as separate. The healing of the splits within the ego has initiated a movement to the periphery that enables the perceptual search for, and recognition of, the good object externally and its representation internally. The presence of the structured remnants of reactions to impingement contributes a differentiating effect.

Splits are maintained beyond stage and phase specificity, when there is an insufficiency of good self-experience. The representations of a whole good self are necessary to provide stability and modulate the traumatic effects of the intensity of biophysiologic demand. When they are deficient, they cannot be structuralized and remain at the interior. A perceptual movement away from that locale would be too disruptive, and the exaggerated need for protection would require that the representations of a bad self be maintained at the periphery. Under these conditions, separation–individuation cannot be successfully negotiated.

The concept of a *basic fault,* as described by Balint (1968), refers to a core of unhealed splits. The basic fault is the equivalent of the effects of that segment on the continuum of instinctual demand that has the qualities of an object that is ominous. This aspect of biophysiologic demand is potentially fragmenting to the self and thereby creates an impression that is represented as a bad instinctual object. The demands of biophysiology are a constant internal source of threat, until sufficient structuralization is attained to maintain a continuous pathway of integration. The effects of this intense source of stimulation on early developmental structures can be modified by the influence of later developments, provided they have not been made defensively inaccessible. The degree to which the impact of biophysiologic demands are increasingly represented, and the basic fault healed, is to a large extent related to the quality of the background object of primary identification. This representation is the background upon which the internalization of perceptual experience takes place, and the firmness of its presence influences the building of all new psychic structures.

The Object Representational System

The mental impressions of those stimuli that elicit body ego experiences are registered and represented as the varied facets of an object's influence. For every quality of experience represented as the self, there is an object-impression counterpart. These object impressions result from perceptual contact with the external world (the object with self-qualities) and from the continuum of biophysiologic demand in the internal world (the self with object qualities).

The initial object impressions, which serve as focal points for good and bad qualities to coalesce, occur at two locales. The first is at the periphery, where perceptual contact with the intrauterine environment has transpired. This impression of a good object's influence is represented as a transitional object and serves as a nidus, which functions to bind the optimally gratifying and optimally frustrating impressions into the representation of a whole good object. The transitional object in the external world possesses attributes that act as an evocative stimulus to this representation and that amplify its containing influence. A transitional object is characterized by residing outside of the self, has qualities of its own that resonate with the experiences of a good object, and functions as a bridge from the self to the object. The fantasy elaboration of this representation forms the transitional space that is necessary as a background, upon which memories and symbolic productions can be anchored. The optimally gratifying impressions are represented as the instinctual aspect of a good object. Initially, phase-specific instinctual gratifications center upon orality and then expand as maturation, the capacity to represent biophysiologic demand, and new body experience advances. This instinctual aspect of a good object follows the progression of the unfolding component instincts.

The second locale is at the interior, where perceptual contact with the continuum of biophysiologic demand takes place. The traumatic-to-unrepresentable dimension of this continuum registers an impression that is ominous, threatening, and possesses instinctual qualities. This powerful, potentially traumatic, instinctual stimulus is experienced as independent of the self and is represented as the instinctual aspect of a bad object. It functions as a nidus around which the object impressions of impingements and deprivations coalesce to form the representation of a whole bad object. This consolidation and organization of the varied impressions of an object's influence into whole entities forms the object representational system. A line of continuity, from the representation of a good to a bad object, is maintained by the shading of optimal frustration (represented in a good object) through prohibitions to impingements (represented in a bad object).

The representation of a transitional object is the object-impression counterpart of the background object of primary identification. Individuals, who have a weak or unstable background object of primary identification, may have an intense need for transitional objects. An overattachment to transitional objects is a manifestation of the effort to compensate for their instability. When the background object of primary identification is solid and firmly established, a transitional object is only utilized during the period of separation–individuation. The transitional object loses its meaning when the object representational system is consolidated, unified, and differentiated. The overextended use of a transitional object may be a reflection of the active presence of the "basic fault" (the traumatic effect of the self with object qualities). The overinvolvement with a transitional object is an attempt to compensate for the internal sense of a threatening presence. There are other individuals, with a faulty background object of primary identification, who experience a transitional object as a threat. Splitting mechanisms abound, separation–individuation has not been negotiated, and the representations of a good object are poorly differentiated. Such individuals will engage in processes of action discharge constantly.

The Process of Separation–Individuation: The Development of the Eye of Consciousness and the Function of Self-Observation

When the representations of good self-experience have been sufficiently structuralized to balance the disruptive effects of biophysiologic demands, the process of separation–individuation is initiated. The intrapsychic manifestation of this development is reflected in a search for the representations of a good object. The continuing consolidation of the representations of good self-experience moves to the periphery. This is the site at which the mental impressions of a good object's influence are coalescing and where the structured remnants of reactions to impingement have remained. It requires a perceptual movement around these reactions to locate the consolidating representations of a good object. The effort and activity exerted to effect this recognition facilitate differentiation, establish the capacity to perceive the good object as separate, and create a new sector of psychological space. The representations of the autonomous ego functions (in the good self) have been extended to perceive the representation of the transitional object (the object-impression counterpart of the background object of primary identification). The effect is to amplify its binding function, add an organizing influence, and facilitate the perception of a separate whole good object. The realm of transitional space that is formed by this expansion of perceptual boundaries is available to contain the mental contents of an evolving system of conscious mental activity.

The body ego experiences of empathic fusion and merger are representations of phase-specific instinctual gratification that transpired in a state of lack of differentiation. When the boundaries of the self expand and locate the representation of a good object, that initial expansion is based on an unstable perception. It is maintained by the exercise of an autonomous ego function and is easily lost under stress or fatigue. Although the perceptual processes are amplified and strengthened by this activity, there is a ready return to the fusion and merger experiences represented and structuralized at the interior. These early stages of self-expansion are unstable, and differentiation is lost and found many times.

The expanding boundaries are extensions of perceptual functioning that have an interior border attuned to the internal world and a peripheral border attuned to the external world. The interior border reflects the influences of the earliest processes of internalization and facilitates the search for the representation of a good object. As this inner perceptual attunement becomes focused, it evolves into the eye of consciousness. This development is at the foundation of the function of self-observation. The peripheral border reflects the influences of the reactions to impingement and fosters the capacity to differentiate the good objects as separate. The structured remnants of reactions to impingement, which remain at the periphery, were based upon a defensive response that necessitated perceptual attunement to the external world. This outer perceptual attunement evolves into a focus of perceptual attention to the stimuli of the external world. The organizational and representational capacities of the far and near receptors are each available to the other because consensual validation has been established. The perceptions of the external world, and of the eye of consciousness in the internal world, have the capacity to evoke the activity of all perceptual modalities. The function of self-observation depends upon the effectiveness with which this developmental milestone is negotiated.

Under conditions in which the representations of good self-experience are deficient, the formation of the eye of consciousness will be tenuous and the function of self-observation faulty. The search for a good object may take place, but almost exclusively in the external world. Although the representations of self-experience may consolidate into good and bad entities, splitting mechanisms are maintained as the major defense of the ego. The representation of a whole good self remains at the interior and a whole bad self at the periphery. This obviates against the discovery of the mental impressions of a good object's influence. The constant disruption at the interior and the ineffective functioning of self-observation create a constant need to find the good object in the external world.

The Development of the First Fixation Point

In a series of sequential steps, the part representations of self-experience form and consolidate into separate entities. A whole good self is organized at the interior and a whole bad self at the periphery, maintaining a connection through a line of continuity of instinctual experience. Their object-impression counterparts are gradually coalescing—the impressions of a good object's influence at the periphery and of a bad object's influence at the interior. A connection is maintained through a line of continuity of prohibitive experience. The structuralization of good self-experience at the interior has initiated the process of separation–individuation, which begins with the healing of the original splits. The continuing representation of good self-experience moves to the periphery, as the representations of bad self-experience recede into the interior. The structured remnants of reactions to impingement remain at the periphery as a differentiating influence. Separation–individuation proceeds with a search for, and location of, the good object and its mental representation, which results in the expansion of self-boundaries. The expanded boundaries of the self have an interior border perceptually attuned to the internal world and a peripheral border perceptually attuned to the external world. Two arms of perception are created. One is an extension of the self-system of representations, as the autonomous ego function of perception moves around the structured remnants of reactions to impingement. I have called this "the introjective arm of perception" because it is the perceptual pathway for external stimuli to evoke the body ego experiences represented in the self. The second reflects the perceptual recognition of the representation of a separate whole good object. I have called this "the projective arm of perception" because it establishes a continuous boundary that enables the evolving system of object representations to be included as a part of the self. It will ultimately serve as the perceptual pathway for projective processes to operate. The interior border has formed a focused area of perceptual activity—the eye of consciousness—and the peripheral border is focused to perceive the stimuli of the outer world.

The emerging function of self-observation has an organizing influence upon the consolidating representations of the good object. This perception of the good object as separate is stabilized by a recognition of its bad qualities. The pathway to that recognition is along the line of continuity of prohibitive experience, which is represented as optimal frustration in the good object and shades through prohibitions into the representation of impingement in the bad object. In this way, the first fixation point forms at the pole of the object representations. It functions to stabilize the newly developed projective arm of perception.

A fixation point will not develop at the introjective arm of perception until the representations of bad self-experience can be recognized. The introjective arm of perception needs to remain open to facilitate the ongoing internalization of interactions with external objects that are necessary for progressive structuralization. The body ego experiences that are represented change with maturational advances and with the increasing capacity for inner regulation, differentiation, and instinctual expansion. The nature of the interactions with external objects that are essential to foster growth must change in accord with these internal developments. The introjective arm of perception, at this stage, must remain open for these processes of internalization to take place. Later, the introjective arm of perception will be stabilized by a recognition of the good self's bad qualities.

Self-expansion occurs in two major ways. The first is manifested in an increasing capacity to represent the demands of biophysiology. In concert with the effects of maturation, the advancing stages of psychosexual development become evident. The representation of instinctual activity gradually expands from oral to anal and later includes phallic and genital dimensions. These stages of psychosexual experience are a product of the interrelationship between the organization and integration of perceptions and perceptual boundaries, expanding contact with the external world of objects and the internal world of biophysiologic demands, and the representation of body ego experiences and their object-impression counterparts. The second major source of self-expansion is through the elaboration in fantasy of each facet of experience, represented in the self and object. These fantasies are then available to serve as a necessary connecting link in the formation of new mental structures. The body ego experiences represented in the self-system and their counterparts, the object impressions represented in the object system, are linked to form the structures that further the progression of separation–individuation and differentiation. The particular linkages that are formed determine the nature and function of the developing structure.

During the period of time that new structures are forming, it is essential for the boundaries of the self to be stabilized. The establishment of this initial fixation point on the projective arm of perception, based on a recognition of the good object's bad qualities, provides that stability. It is then possible for new structures to evolve that will unite and differentiate the two systems of representation.

The Formation of New Structure

The effect of the perceptual recognition of the separateness of the object is of an intense experience of helplessness and vulnerability. This is potentially traumatic and creates the need to achieve a balance for that disturbing perception. A motive is present to utilize the available mental representations in an adaptive fashion and further the thrust for continuing differentiation. This shift toward inner regulation is accomplished by the formation of a new structure, which can function to unite and differentiate the self- and object systems of representation (and alleviate the experience of vulnerability).

The recognition of separateness occurs during the height of the anal period. Instinctual body ego experiences and their object impressions have expanded along the lines of psychosexual development and are represented according to their good and bad qualities in the self and object. Instinctual body ego experiences of regulation and control do not require defense and are represented in the good self. Instinctual body ego experiences of anal sadism (poorly neutralized libidinal and aggressive drives) require defense and are represented in the bad self. The impression of a good instinctual object is represented as one providing optimal opportunities for mastery, and of a bad instinctual object as anally sadistic. Each aspect, represented in the self and object, is elaborated in fantasy. The fantasies are then accessible to serve as the linkages by which connections are established. The recognition of separateness has occurred at the periphery, the site at which the representations of a whole good self and good object are organizing. These representations of good qualities of experience are particularly suitable for the stage- and phase-specific needs that have evolved.

The experience of helplessness and vulnerability is balanced by the formation of a new structure that enables the self to participate in the fantasied omnipotence of the object. It is for this reason that I have called it the "grandiose self." (Throughout the literature, there has been much confusion as to the origin, fate, composition, and function of the grandiose self. There has also been confusion as to the process by which wishful self-images are transformed into realistic self-images. I hope to bring some clarity to these questions in the course of this exposition.) The fixation point on the projective arm of perception has provided the necessary stability, and the formation of this new structure is initiated by the good instinctual aspect of self-experience's seeking an attachment to the representation of a good object. In health, this transpires during the anal phase when control, mastery, and autonomy are in the ascendency. The instinctual representation of a good object is elaborated into a fantasy of omnipotence, which is a perfect antidote for the vulnerability of separateness. This fantasy provides the link that structurally unites and differentiates the two systems of representation at the periphery. The good instinctual aspect of the self is linked to the good instinctual aspect of the object, through a fantasy of omnipotence, to form the structure of the grandiose self.

The creation of the grandiose self occupies a significant segment of good instinctual self-experience with maintaining a fantasy. Until it is firmly structured, it has the effect of weakening the whole good self (represented at the periphery) in its adaptive functions. A need is elicited to strengthen the self-representational system, which motivates the formation of another new structure. Primitive identifications, occurring through fusion–merger experiences in a state of lack of differentiation, have enabled the influences of an object to facilitate, amplify, and expand the representations of self-experience. In the more advanced level of psychic organization that has now been achieved, the process of identification is more selective and discriminating and is invoked with the internal representation of the object. The second new structure that is formed at the periphery strengthens the good self-representations through selective identification, and further unites and differentiates the two systems of representation. The representations of the autonomous ego functions in the good self are elaborated in fantasy and link to the admired qualities represented in the object. The qualities most admired in the object will be determined by what is most deficient in the self. For this reason, I have called this structure the "ego ideal."

The particular body ego experiences and their object impressions that have been represented and elaborated in fantasy determine the composition of these differentiating structures. They evolve as a mental substrate that has a strong influence upon the emerging process of symbolization. Their composition highlights the qualities in an interaction that facilitate growth and those that are an interference. The grandiose self and ego ideal lay the groundwork for what will later appear as a hierarchy of organization for the id of the dynamic unconscious. These unifying and differentating structures provide a framework that reflects the beginning stages of superego organization and the onset of cohesiveness within the self. The tripartite structures of id, ego, and superego can only become functional when cohesiveness is firmly secured. The formation of the grandiose self and ego ideal increases the range of experiences that are available for representation, fosters integrative functions, enhances differentiation, and strengthens autonomy.

The developmental experience of a male, and of a female, will differ as a consequence of the differences in body ego experience. For example, the body ego experience of genital exploration in a boy will be entirely different than that in a girl. A girl exploring the hidden, unseen recesses of her body has an entirely different attitude toward the process of inner exploration. A girl will have more difficulty in differentiating some areas of body ego experience (the anal and vaginal area are very close to each other anatomically, by innervation and by sensation). These differences are reflected in the representations of self-experience, their object-impression counterparts, and in the fantasy elaborations that function as linkages in structure building. Their significance will be considered when discussing later stages in development, when they are more noticeable.

These descriptions have centered upon healthy development and only hinted at the pathological potentialities. The events portrayed here are descriptive of a healthy grandiose self and ego ideal. In pathology, they can develop in a distorted fashion.

The Interrelationship between Perception and Structure Formation

The expanded boundaries of the self have an interior border with a focused area of perceptual activity (the eye of consciousness) and a peripheral border with a focused area of perceptual activity (the perceptions of the external world). These borders are an extension of two aspects of self-experience. One has involved a search in the interior for the representation of a good object. The other has involved the anticipation of impingements from the external world. The two focused areas of perception consolidate at the point of contact with the external world. The interior focus has evolved into the eye of consciousness, which functions to look inward and observe the mental contents of the conscious system. The peripheral focus functions to look outward and receive immediate perceptual impressions.

When the boundaries of the self expand to include the representations of the object, the formation of differentiating structures is made possible. The process of establishing linkages requires the function of perception, and the interior and peripheral borders are incorporated as the grandiose self and ego ideal are created. The grandiose self is an instinctual structure that necessitated the location of a good instinctual object's influence. The interior border, attuned to such an internal search, is especially suited to determining that pathway. The ego ideal is based upon selective identifications that are motivated by deficiencies in the self-system of representations. The fantasy elaboration of autonomous functions seek an attachment to the admired qualities of an object's influence. The peripheral border, attuned to perceptions of an external object, is especially suited to determine that pathway.

The grandiose self and ego ideal possess perceptual borders with the identical capacities developed at the point of contact with the external world. I have called this internal agency of perception the "superego eye." The interior border, encompassing the grandiose self and developing a focus of perceptual attention to the interior, is capable of perceiving the contents of the deeper layers of preconscious mental activity. The peripheral border, encompassing the ego ideal and developing an outward focus of perceptual attention, is capable of perceiving the contents of conscious mental activity (that which is perceived by the eye of consciousness from a different perspective).

In the state of dreaming, perceptions are registered primarily by the superego eye. The perceptual functioning of the eye of consciousness and the immediate perceptions of the external world are in a state of suspension or limited activity. The perceptions registered by the superego eye will be predominantly of the instinctual derivatives evoked by the activity of the id of the dynamic unconscious. The dreamer's experience will be directed by this more regressive, less well-developed perceptual focus. In dreams, the boundaries of the self are determined by the superego eye, and the contents of the conscious system are perceived as outside of the self.

The interior border is involved in the formation of, and is regulated by, the grandiose self. This perceptual border is an integral part of a structure based on fantasy and readily follows the dominance of the pleasure principle. Condensations and displacements, which occur in the unconscious system, affect the mental contents in the preconscious system. The fluid shifts of perceptual attention that are thereby required are readily regulated by the grandiose self. The peripheral border is involved in the formation of, and regulated by, the ego ideal. This perceptual border is an integral part of a structure based on identifications and readily follows the dominance of the reality principle. The mental contents of the conscious system are logical, sequential, and occupied by memory traces of immediate perceptions and by symbolic thought and language. The stable focus of perceptual attention that is required is readily regulated by the ego ideal.

Mental contents, which are linear, logical, sequential, and filled with immediate perceptions, are a product of the activity of the eye of consciousness. They do not offer direct access to the derivatives reflective of unconscious mental activity. It is essential to have a grasp of those conditions that foster a suspension of this perceptual activity, so as to allow the perceptual activity of the superego eye to assert itself.

Discussion

As *A* became verbally communicative, he was able to describe his inner experiences. It became possible to achieve a deeper understanding of the composition of his representational world. Very early in the therapeutic contact, his behavior appeared to be a manifestation of his disengagement from the external world of stimuli and of the impact of powerful forces attacking him from within. He began to verbalize his experiences, and the nature of these forces became more explicable. Instinctual demands constantly exerted their effects upon his perceptual processes, which were reflected in the shifting representations of the Make-A-Dos. These instinctual figures ranged from being fun-loving, pleasurable, and not requiring defense, to becoming frightening and requiring defense, to escalating in size as an ominous and dangerous presence. The concept of an original impingement at the interior, in response to the demands of biophysiology, appeared to be verified. They appeared as a constant source of instinctual activity that *A* was attempting to integrate and defend against. The impinging qualities of these instinctual representations were distinguishable from the impingements of the external world. These object impressions of external impingements were represented with differing characteristics that were revealing. They were portrayed in the figures of the Big Black Pops and The Big Pain, which had prohibitive qualities and were patterned after parental interactions. The powerful impact of these internal and external stimuli affected the manner in which the self was represented. This was reflected in the image of Pa-Ba—a split-off, passive, damaged, and shapeless infant.

There was little evidence in these representations, or in the observations of his behavior, of an inner experience of vulnerability and helplessness. *A* might convey this appearance to the observer but gave little indication of such a feeling state within himself. Even the figure of Pa-Ba, the one representation that might imply such a feeling state, had no definition, shape, or form. Pa-Ba was a totally subjugated, depleted, and shapeless self, hardly capable of any feeling state.

The therapeutic relationship continued, and *A* began to indicate the manner in which he was representing that interaction. This was evidenced in his increasing capacity to communicate and in the emergence of a new representational figure: the soldier. *A*'s ability to form an attachment to the therapist was paralleled by the evolution of this mental representation. The previously split-off, fragmented representations of good self-experience consolidated into a whole, in response to unconsciously empathic interactions. These interactions created object impressions with a quality of goodness that was embodied in the representation of the soldier.

A, in molding himself to the body of the therapist, seemed to be experiencing a symbiotic state of lack of differentiation. In that state, the effects of the interaction could be internalized. The experience of the self-seeking gratification and of an object's offering comfort and containment seemed to be blurred, indistinct, and fluctuating. The representation of these indistinct and shifting experiences appeared to be forming in conjunction with his molding behavior. The therapist sensed an unconscious message reflecting the inner need for qualities of optimal frustration to amplify his latent and developing functional abilities. The therapist, in both words and behavior, expressed the idea of wanting A to be a functional separate individual. The effect was to invoke an awareness in A of his separateness from the therapist. It was at this point that A seemed to experience an inner feeling of vulnerability and helplessness. This had also transpired on the eve of an interruption caused by the therapist's vacation.

The representations of good self-experience could only consolidate when the therapeutic interaction was empathic to A's unconscious communications, and initially this appeared to take place in the interior. The disruptive impact of biophysiologic demand, as reflected in the ominous aspect of the Make-A-Dos, became modulated. The representations of a whole good self gradually became more firmly established and, as they did, were more in evidence and accessible at the periphery (the point of contact with the external world). Concurrently, the impressions of a good object's influence were organizing and consolidating in the image of the soldier. The splits in the self were healing, manifested by psychic functioning that necessitated a consolidation of the representations of good self-experience into a unified entity. The splits in the ego were also healing, manifested by the evidence of their functioning at the periphery. The consequence was in A's being more accessible to the interpretive interventions of the therapist. Correspondingly, the representations of bad self-experience that had dominated A's reactions to external stimuli appeared to recede into the interior.

The emergence of A's recognition of the separateness of the therapist was associated with a profound feeling of helplessness and vulnerability. The therapist's departure invoked a return to the previously established union with the Make-A-Dos. The representations of a good self and good object, developing in response to the therapeutic interaction, were tenuous and insufficiently stabilized to be effectively maintained without the reinforcement of continuing contact. However, they remained internalized, ready to be called forth when conditions were present that supported their functioning.

The return of the therapist, and the potential for reestablishing contact, immediately evoked these representations of the therapeutic interaction. A's response was to relinquish his attachment to his bodily products. The therapist's immediate reaction was empathically attuned to these inner events. However, the conflicts engendered by this empathic resonance elicited a defensive reaction in the therapist that impinged upon A. The therapist became a parallel of the impinging object impressions that had been so prevalent in A's internal world. The effect was to disrupt the consolidating representations of good self-experience that had been evolving and to reinstitute the protective armor of an autistic withdrawal. The influence of fragmented part self- and part object configurations dominated the interaction, as the earlier splits in the self and in the ego reasserted themselves.

The therapist gradually gained an understanding of what had transpired. He was able to express his understanding in words and behavior, and specifically, to acknowledge the part he played in this traumatic interaction. It was only then that A slowly began to communicate the effects it had upon him. As he did so, the representations of good self-experience became more consolidated, organized, and stabilized at the interior, and the healing of splits in the ego resurfaced. The process of separation–individuation was in evidence once again, and A's experience of vulnerability re-emerged.

A period of lack of differentiation was required for the effects of the therapeutic interaction to be internalized and be available to form representational structures. Empathically responsive interactions evoked body ego experiences represented within the good self and left object impressions represented as a good object.

Initially, the representations of self-experience were in a fragmented, underdeveloped state. It required a long period of sustained empathic responsiveness for the state of lack of differentiation to be manifested. When the representations of a whole good self had been sufficiently consolidated, the process of separation–individuation could gradually be instigated. It was necessary for the therapist to provide the qualities of optimal frustration and to amplify the seeds of autonomous functioning that initiated the individuating process. The point at which the separateness of the self and object was recognized was associated with the experience of helplessness and vulnerability.

E was a child whose level of personality organization was quite advanced. He was well into forming an intense oedipal conflict, which was interfering with further developmental progression. He had negotiated the early process of separation–individuation, established cohesiveness, and was forming the object-related perceptual capacities associated with genital expansion. The residual effects of his early infantile attachment to a maternal figure had influenced each succeeding level of advancement. This infantile attachment exerted a regressive pull with each new conflict engendered by advances in development.

Early in the therapeutic contact, he maintained a perception of the therapist that fostered his integrative processes. The therapist, in turn, had maintained an attitude responsive to his unconscious communications. The interaction embodied the therapist as a container of E's productions. The therapist functioned to metabolize E's psychic experiences and return them to him in the form of interpretive comments. E internalized the interpretations and utilized them to more effectively integrate his inner psychic contents. The intensity of instinctual demand heightened, defensive responses became more active, and E exerted interactional pressure upon the therapist to reinforce his character defenses. The therapist's participation was perceived by E as a repetition of his transference anticipations. The therapist eventually recognized and acknowledged the part he played in this transference reenactment. The therapist's recognition was also reflected in his behavior so that the lapse in unconscious empathy could be rectified. This was a crucial dimension in E's ability to perceive the transference distortion.

At this point, the powerful stimulus of his mother's pregnancy evoked an active return of the representational structures that reflected his experience with separation and individuation. *E* could feel the intense pull to be close to a maternal figure, which eroded his functional capacities. *E*'s fantasy of the pile of snow with the tunnel frozen over, from which he could only emerge by forcing himself through the roof, was particularly interesting. *E* had been the product of a caesarian birth. The impact of that body ego experience on later mental representations and their elaboration in fantasy were striking. The movement of forcing himself to escape from an enclosed space also reflected his characteristic manner of responding to regressive infantile longing.

E began to experience the feeling of helplessness and vulnerability associated with separateness, and his character structure motivated him to exert interactional pressure upon the therapist to reinforce its defensive functions. He was unconsciously concerned that the therapist would again respond defensively and be experienced as a seductive and provocative figure. The therapist's recognition of this anxiety and of the earlier part he had played in repeating the trauma gave *E* the inner experience of being unconsciously understood. His derivative associations reflected his wish to be separate and to find qualities of goodness in varying interactions. He was then able to experience the vulnerability of separateness. He indicated the presence of a structure that provided balance for this inner sense of helplessness and vulnerability. It consisted of the self, represented as capable of mastery and control, linked through a fantasy of the object's omnipotence to the representation of a gratifying object. This attachment allowed *E* to participate in the object's omnipotent qualities and reflected the manner in which the grandiose self had formed. He spoke of his mother's having the best things to give and of leaving her goodness to go off on his own. He could balance his vulnerability by carrying the fantasy of omnipotence with him.

The potential dangers, which *E* anticipated in being separate, gave expression to the depletion created by maintaining this structure. It was followed by a shift to elaborating his potentials in fantasy, which reflected the functioning of the ego ideal. *E*'s fantasies were linked to admired qualities of masculine effectiveness, expressive of selective identifications that strengthened his self system.

The potentials of the self were elaborated in fantasy and linked to those admired qualities represented in the object that were most needed. *E*'s shift to elaborating his heroic abilities involved the qualities he admired most in his father and reinforced his masculine identifications.

CHAPTER 5

The Onset of Cohesiveness

The Formation and Function of the Grandiose Self and the Ego Ideal

Introduction

It is often assumed, either implicitly or explicitly, that every mental activity has meaning. It is certainly true that any particular psychological experience, or mode of adaptation to the stimuli of the internal and external worlds, reflects the functioning of healthy or pathological structures. Mental activities, no matter what their nature, do have the potential of providing information that can lend itself to a deeper understanding of an individual. I believe it is inaccurate to extend this idea to the assumption that every mental production or psychological experience has meaning. Therefore, I would like to offer a definition of meaning that can lend itself to a determination of when meaning is present and when it is absent.

Mental representations of body ego experiences and object impressions are all elaborated in fantasies, which function as connecting links. Meaning is produced by the linkage of the representations of self-experience to the object impressions that have elicited them. All three elements must be present for meaning to result. Defined in this way, linkages are established as the vehicle for the production of meaning. The destruction of, or nonproduction of, linkages leads to the destruction of, or nonproduction of, meaning. The destruction of meaning can occur in all realms of mental activity and depends upon the process involved in its destruction. Meaning can be destroyed by suppression and a conscious refusal to fantasize, by defensive opposition to fantasy that is unconsciously determined, or by the lack of development of fantasy elaborations.

In listening to patients for a determination of meaning, we may lose sight of the fact that each individual speaks and listens from every aspect of his or her unique character. If we only consider one aspect of character in our understanding, we do not understand at all. If we look only at the projective aspect of an individual's communications, we may understand it and even understand it accurately. However, if the introjective aspect of communicaiton and the connecting linkage has not been seen, the person has not been understood. The introjective aspect refers to the unconscious perceptions of the therapist's activities, silences, and interpretations. To look only at the fantasied projections of these experiences is to miss the context in which they occur. It ignores the adaptive significance of that context and the unconscious direction as to how a cure can best take place. The therapist, in not listening to this aspect of the patient's experience, may unwittingly participate in the destruction of meaning. To see transference only as a projection fosters an interaction in which the establishment of meaning is undermined.

Another factor, which is often involved in eroding meaning, is the assumption that everything has meaning. This assumption can interfere with the process of creating conditions in which meaning can be experienced. What, then, is the experience of that which has no meaning? There are several possibilities: body ego experiences without fantasy elaborations or connections to object imagery, object impressions without the associated body ego experiences, or isolated fantasy elaborations. Isolated fantasy elaborations can be present as psychic content, due to the effects of repressive or suppressive defensive activity. An awareness of the absence of meaning makes it possible to determine how it has been destroyed and, in turn, how it can be restored.

Ultimately, meaning is destroyed by the effects of defensive activity. When the primary stimulus resides in the therapeutic interaction, it must be identified, rectified, and interpreted. Only then can the underlying foundation of a given psychological experience be illuminated, for a determination of the presence or absence of meaning. For example, a patient may complain of some difficulty in a relationship and only present the feeling of hurt, anger, rejection, or disappointment. The therapist, aware of the missing fantasies, may confront the patient with their absence. The confrontation is experienced as a criticism or attack, which mobilizes defensive reactions to the impingement. Conversely, the therapist may chose to empathize with the patient's conscious feeling, which directs attention away from the missing fantasies. The therapist may decide to listen in silence until the patient can communicate further. The patient may then ask questions or express the need for a response. The therapist, having historical material available, may offer an interpretation as to the genetic determinants of the complaint. This type of intervention says to a patient, "When you turn to me and begin to bring the missing fantasies, expressed in your behavior and questions, I will present you a communicative message that directs attention away from what offers a potential for meaning and toward that which reinforces the destruction of meaning." The therapist has provided a logical, orderly thought that directs perceptual attention to the conscious system and away from the area of derivative expressions where linkages are formed and developed. These aforementioned forms of interaction would foster a mode of communication that tended to be devoid of meaning.

Derivatives, by their nature, include all of the elements that define meaning. There is a body ego experience that is represented, elaborated into a fantasy, and linked to its object-impression counterpart. Patients with inner cohesiveness and structural organization communicate more meaning. Efforts to destroy meaning and invite the therapist's participation in its destruction are more easily seen by both parties as a defensive function. In primitively organized, narcissistic personalities, the absence of meaning is an aspect of communication that is a part of the pathology itself. Healthy structures are so unstable that they are vulnerable to destruction, in any but the most unconsciously empathic type of interaction. Such individuals may test the climate of a therapeutic relationship by presenting communications devoid of meaning. The therapist who treats these communications as meaningful reveals an unawareness of meaning and, hence, is experienced as a potential source of danger. The lack of recognition is perceived as having destructive intent.

Individuals are often selective in their heightened sensitivity and accurate in perceiving the therapist's unconscious motivation for this lack of recognition. It may involve a therapist's unconscoius fear of the regression that a particular interaction potentially engenders. In addition, therapists are often trained to believe that everything has meaning. This may be difficult to unlearn. The presence of mental content alone does not signify meaning. When a primitively organized patient communicates with meaning, it is a very frightening experience. It is essential that an atmosphere be created wherein such communications can take place in relative safety. A significant ingredient of that atmosphere concerns the therapist's ability to recognize what is, and what is not, meaningful. A patient who has had the experience very early in life of a relationship that resulted in the destruction of meaning is in a position where that which is needed threatens self-destruction. For healing to occur, this process needs once again to be activated in a relationship. It is fraught with danger when the therapeutic partner in the relationship does not recognize the structure and function of meaning.

An understanding of development processes establishes a theoretical basis for discriminating healthy from pathological forms of communication and for understanding the foundation of projective and introjective mechanisms. Therapeutic interventions are guided by a patient's reactions and responses. The validity and significance of an interpretation is determined by the imagery that is evoked. It is essential to have available a background knowledge as to what constitutes the derivative expression of a healthy, and a pathological, relationship. It is precisely at that critical point in development when the individual is emerging from the lack of differentiation embodied in a psychological symbiosis that there is a capacity to establish the mental representational foundation for the expression of derivatives. The symbiosis has been necessary to enable the internalization, representation, and consolidation of good and bad self-experiences. When these are sufficiently consolidated, differentiation proceeds. Cohesiveness is initiated when the representations of an object are perceived as separate and new unifying and differentiating mental structures are formed. The production of meaning is dependent upon the effective functioning of these intrapsychic structures.

In previous chapters, I presented a theoretical construct to illuminate the original body ego experience that underlies, and provides a foundation for, the process of internalization. In the absence of such a concept, the developmental line for an experience originating outside of the self and becoming a part of the self is incomplete. In this chapter, I will enlarge upon its significance and review the early developmental events leading up to and including the process of separation–individuation. I will also review, and further discuss, the new psychic structures that are formed to maintain differentiation and the functions that evolve from them. The negotiation of this developmental step is essential for the production of meaning. I will then present a brief portrayal of the significance of these events for establishing the necessary preconditions for the evolution of an oedipal conflict.

Clinical Material

A tentatively and cautiously reestablished a connection to the therapist. It was manifested in the return of his capacity to verbally communicate his inner experiences. For the first time, *A* began to test the boundaries and limits of the therapist. He was also testing the depth of the therapist's understanding of the previous rupture that had been so traumatic for him. He spent the ensuing months, at first cautiously and then with more intensity, searching for objects in the room that he could attempt to destroy: knocking over a lamp, attempting to break a statue, and so on. He established a scenario that could be interpreted as an expression of hostility but appeared to be probing to see if the therapist would recognize that he was seeking maternal and containing responses. He apparently had recreated a microcosm of the previous trauma. The therapist's first response was to let *A* know that he did not want him to hurt the objects in his room. *A* anxiously proceeded to attack these objects, and the therapist gently held and contained him. The therapist experienced these interactions as a means of forming a bond of closeness. It felt to the therapist like he was comforting a very young child who was exploring his capacity to affect the external environment.

A gradually began to talk about events in his life and to elaborate them in fantasy. It was the first time that he had spoken of varied individuals and situations. He described interactions with his mother, father, brother, and other children. The world of objects represented in his mind was proliferating. The quality of the interactions he described involved his efforts to attain some measure of mastery of his environment at home and school. He spoke of his frustrations and anxiety and of an upsurge of anger. He was particularly fearful at these moments. He began to develop a fantasy in which *A* and the therapist were special agents who possessed special skills and abilities and could succeed at any task. *A* was a special agent whose task was to secure knowledge of other people and institutions. He would find obstacles to attaining that knowledge and be seen as an enemy who must be thwarted or from whom knowledge was hidden. *A* would then consult with the therapist, who was the head of the special agents. *A* and the therapist would then work together to figure out what the obstacle or frustration was and find a way to overcome it. *A* delighted in this fantasy. He became totally absorbed when the therapist would say, "Well, that's a tough one; let's think about it and see what we know and can figure out." *A* would excitedly participate in presenting the information he had, sharing it with the therapist, and then both would search for a solution.

The following session occurred after *A* had learned that he would be separated from the therapist for a week. He was going to a long-planned family reunion in a distant city. *A* began the session by telling the therapist about the trip. He was going on an airplane. He began to express his extreme anxiety that the plane would not get off the ground or would crash. He very anxiously repeated questions to the therapist as to whether that could happen—"Could the plane crash? Will it fly?" The therapist stated that he thought *A* was extremely fearful that in being separate from the therapist he would be unable to fly on his own and be unable to carry an image of the therapist that would allow him to be separate and remain whole. *A* then had the idea that as Special Agent X-9 he could enter the airplane, learn about it, see if it was safe, see how it flew, and learn its secrets. He could see if there were any troubles and report them to the pilot of the plane. The plane could then take off and fly. If the pilot would not listen to him or would ignore him, it would let A know not to fly on that airplane. He then began to worry about the trip back. He might trust the pilot who brought him there, but if he could not trust the pilot who brought him back, he would be left in a distant place. The therapist stated that he thought A was reminding him of the previous occasion when there had been an interruption; there had been a crash when he returned. The therapist had not been the trustworthy pilot he had been when he left. The therapist thought A was worried it would happen again. A then talked of his family at the reunion and specifically of his grandfather. He knew him well. He looked forward to seeing him. On the evening following this session, the therapist received a telephone call from A at the airport. He stated simply, "This is Special Agent X-9 reporting the airplane is OK."

F was a 9-year-old boy referred because of poor school performance, temper tantrums when faced with any frustration, and his constant complaint of hating himself. He was extremely conforming and submissive at home and wild and uncontrollable in school. F was eager to see a therapist, and from the beginning, sat quietly in a chair and was extremely verbal. He spoke rapidly with no pauses. He talked of his unhappiness and hatred of himself: he felt he was bad, angry, and enraged. He wanted to see the therapist regularly, and often, to talk about his troubles. Therapy began, and F talked uninterruptedly from the beginning to the end of his sessions. He barely paused to get his breath and continued on with a new narrative. He described interactions with other children that focused on mischief, getting away with breaking rules, fooling teachers, and engaging in horseplay out of sight of authorities. When the therapist reflected upon his preoccupation with getting away with things and fooling authorities and wondered if these thoughts expressed his experience with the therapist, F immediately protested that it had nothing to do with his therapy. He welcomed and valued the experience and felt free to talk about these hidden activities. This was the only place he could talk about them. He then went on to describe the prohibiting, inhibiting, controlling nature of his home environment. He had to be polite and conforming at all times. He had to dress properly and call parental figures Sir and Ma'am. It was a welcome relief to be talking with the therapist where that was not necessary. He could reveal his playfulness and mischievousness. He was terrified of his father's anger at home and thus had to be the model of politeness. Here he was not afraid. He continued to fill the hours with tales of his mischief. After some time, these tales were interspersed with complaints about being treated unfairly by his parents. This centered on his relationship with his siblings. F was the oldest of four and felt he was the scapegoat. The other children could do anything, and he was expected to be responsible for what they did. Any trouble was always his fault. This made him feel bad about himself. In his parents' eyes, he could do nothing well. The therapist attempted to relate these complaints to his feeling unfairly treated by the therapist. F again protested that these complaints had nothing to do with the therapist.

After many months, the therapist noticed that he was feeling lost and bewildered in his efforts to understand F. Although F was eager to come and filled the hours with a plethora of verbal productions, the therapist had no inner feeling of being connected to F. On the surface, the things he talked about appeared to be expressing his inner thoughts and feelings. However, the therapist noted that he had learned nothing new from F in the material he communicated. It was a seemingly endless repetition of his episodes of mischief and fooling authorities or of his complaints of mistreatment and scapegoating at the hands of his parents. For a period of time, the therapist was drawn to linear interpretive statements; that is, the therapist commented on F's difficulties with managing his aggression, on his envy of siblings, or at one point interpreting F's productions as covering his anxiety over sexual feelings. F responded to these comments in a surprising way. First, he stated, "I think you are right; I hadn't thought of that before." He then elaborated on the therapist's comment by adding, "I was more angry than I realized" or "I guess I really do envy my brother and sister" or "I don't like to think about sexual things." He then went on to repeat anew the same themes and narratives.

The therapist began to notice that in all of F's productions, there was always a missing ingredient. When he spoke of relationships, his focus was on the actions and responses of others. He left out his inner reactions and feeling states. At other times, he spoke of his inner feeling states but left out the fantasy or the responses of others. Periodically, he described isolated fantasies with no apparent connection to a context that had elicited them. The following session occurred as the therapist was struggling to understand the significance of these observations.

F began by speaking, in his characteristic fashion, of a series of events in school wherein he had either tricked, fooled, or out-witted the teacher. The therapist listened and thought of it as a derivative expression of what F was doing with the therapist. The therapist also recalled that in the past, when he had attempted to address this communication, it was immediately denied by F. The therapist thought that somehow he had not created an environ-ment in which F felt safe enough to reveal what was inside of him and found it necessary to engage in a constant effort to keep him-self hidden. The therapist then spoke in an effort to communicate this thought to F. As the therapist's words were expressed, they became jumbled and were spoken in a confusing manner. The therapist became acutely aware that his words were hardly under-standable, paused to explore his inner reactions, and tried to de-termine what had affected him. When he paused, F began to talk, "I see what you mean." F then expressed the idea that he was validating the therapist's observation. The impact of that moment struck the therapist. He took in F's words, "I see what you mean," in a different way. F saw that the therapist's words had no mean-ing. The therapist became aware that this was exactly the ex-perience he was having with F. F's words were having no meaning to the therapist. The therapist had been feeling much discomfort in participating in an interaction where no meaning was expressed. The therapist then communicated his realization to F. He thought F was pointing out that the therapist's words had no meaning. F was calling the therapist's attention to how much this had predominated in the course of their experience together. There was a long silence. F appeared uneasy and embarrassed. He squirmed and began to talk. As he sat in the chair, it was as if there were two of him. One was in the forefront talking to the therapist and telling him whatever he could think of to say. Another part of him was sitting far back in the chair observing the therapist. He watched the therapist's reactions, listened to his words, watched what he responded to and to what he did not, and observed his facial expressions. Way in the back of his mind, he wondered what the therapist wanted from him or expected of him. He was constantly weighing what would or would not elicit the therapist's approval. F had a deep inner feeling that he did not know how to talk from this part of himself to the therapist. As he was talking now, he had the feeling that this part of himself was the most important of all. He felt very distrustful of everyone around him and of the therapist. His whole manner of being and his entire manner of interacting were based upon the way he had been talking to the therapist. He now had a feeling that maybe he could really talk for the first time. He described how small and insignificant he felt. He was overwhelmed by the demands of school, his parents, and of the whole world that surrounded him. He felt ineffective, inadequate, and vulnerable to the attacks and words of others. He felt distant, isolated and separate. It felt like no one could really reach him. He commented on the sound of his voice and became tearful. It was the first time he could hear the sound of his own voice. He turned to the therapist and spoke of his recognition that the therapist was confused by him and lost in attempting to understand him. He wondered often how the therapist could listen to his words and not be able to somehow hear him and help him to be able to talk. Today was the first time he could talk. It reminded him of a story he read in which a young prince had been cursed and had to live a life of isolation and ugliness. He could only be rescued by someone having the capacity to see the prince hidden in the ugliness.

The Self with Object Qualities

With the dawning of sensory perceptual processes, the effects of interactions with the external world and of biophysiologic demand in the internal world are registered. The latent capacity of the primitive ego for mental representation is awakened, and an initial, primitive reactive state of consciousness is created. These original body ego experiences are at the foundation of all further mental development, and the manner in which the stimuli are represented determines the boundaries of a nuclear self. An ongoing interrelationship is gradually established between the perceptual processes and the representational functions of the ego.

The demands of biophysiology present a continuing source of stimulation, emanating from the interior of the organism. These stimuli are registered by the perceptual processes, but their variability and intensity are such that they are represented as having different qualities.

One element on the continuum of biophysiological demand elicits a body ego experience that can be contained within the boundaries of the nuclear self without the need for defense. This instinctual experience is represented as a facet of the good self (the nidus for phase-specific instinctual gratifications). Another element is overstimulating and contained with the aid of defense. This instinctual experience is represented as a facet of the bad self. A further element cannot be fully contained within the boundaries of the nuclear self but is registered as a mental impression with the independent characteristics of an object. This instinctual object impression is represented as a facet of the bad object (the nidus around which the representations of external impingements and deprivations will coalesce). There is also an element on the continuum of biophysiological demand that is incapable of being registered by the perceptual processes. This dimension possesses all of the qualities of an object and, though part of the organism, remains outside of the self. I have called this entire continuum of biophysiological demand, "the self with object qualities," as stated previously. It offers a concept to illuminate the status of the nuclear self and the original body ego experience that is available as a foundation for the internalization of the effects of perceptual contact with the intrauterine world.

There is much evidence to suggest that the onset of perceptual functioning takes place *in utero*. This is the first perceptual contact with the external world, and it is occurring in conjunction with the body ego experiences that are evolving from perceptual contact with the self with object qualities in the internal world. The physiologic, metabolic, buffering functions of the maternal intrauterine environment are registered concurrently with the stimuli of biophysiological demand. The body ego experience is of a containing interaction, simultaneously, inside and outside of the nuclear self. It is represented as the background object of primary identification and serves as the original object of libidinal demand. It is in this way that an element of biophysiologic demand can be registered and represented without defense. The conditions necessary as a mental substrate for processes of internalization to be functional are unfolding in this primitive state of perception. A psychological symbiosis in postuterine life can only be created when the external world is capable of sufficient empathic resonance to evoke and amplify this basic foundation.

The Object with Self-Qualities

The original ego is a body ego under the dominance of the reality principle. The nucleus of autonomy is, at its foundation, a core of the nuclear self that is objectless. In a very primitive way, there is an original sense of separateness, as the newborn infant reactively experiences the self and the nonself as different. This body ego experience functions as the core upon which all further self-differentiation builds.

The representation of the background object of primary identification has required perceptual contact with an object (the intrauterine environment). This contact occurs under conditions that are characterized by a lack of differentiation and results in a body ego experience that is represented as a facet of the good self. It is present within the nuclear self as the original object for the representation of libidinal demand. Libido is conceptualized as object seeking, which means that instinctual gratification depends upon the presence of an object's influence and cannot take place in an objectless state. The physiologic, metabolic functions of the intrauterine environment are registered as simultaneously inside and outside of the nuclear self (that is, an object with self-qualities).

When the external object is empathically responsive to the conditions of the newborn infant's internal world, it evokes and amplifies the representation of the background object of primary identification. The core of objectless experience recedes into the background, as the fusion–merger experiences of lack of differentiation predominate. This symbiotic interaction is necessary to internalize the influence of a good object and elicit the body ego experiences and object impressions upon which further development depends. Optimally gratifying activities expand the experience of phase-specific instinctual gratification. The optimally frustrating aspects of the interaction amplify the exercise of autonomous functions. The restraint involved in optimal frustration readily extends to periods of prohibition and impingement, and there are inevitable sensory deprivations. When in proportion, these latter qualities facilitate differentiation and enable the effectiveness of defense. I have called this continuum of an external object's influence, as stated before, the object with self-qualities. There is an element that is experienced as a part of the self, an element that is enhancing to the autonomous functioning of the self, and an element that is independent and necessitates defense.

The body ego experiences and object impressions of perceptual contact with the self with object qualities at the interior foster internalization of the effects of perceptual contact with the object with self-qualities at the periphery. This process of internalization increases the capacity to represent the demands of biophysiology. In conjunction with maturation, each progressive developmental step is dependent upon and affected by the step that has preceded it. Thus interferences in early development will have the most profound and debilitating effects. The particular nature of the pathology has embedded in it the sequences of development that have been affected and the potential for revealing a pathway to its cure. For example, the pathway to the cure of autism is in the formation of a healthy symbiosis. Autistic pathology reveals the results of an inadequate symbiosis.

The Expansion of the Self- and Object Representations into Functional Systems

The varied representations of part self-experience and their object-impression counterparts are initially localized where the impact of their stimuli has been registered. The mechanism of splitting facilitates their coalescence, in accordance with their good and bad qualities, where they are most needed. There are particular aspects that highlight the quality and nature of the experience and serve as a nidus to facilitate the consolidation of parts into unified entities.

The background object of primary identification is initially represented at the interior, where its containing influence buffers the disruptive effect of biophysiologic demand. At this site, it is most acceptable for enabling the continuing expansion of good self-experience through instinctual representation. It serves as the nidus around which all aspects of good self-experience consolidate. The reactions to impingement are initially represented at the periphery, where their differentiating influence balances the lack of differentiation embodied in a psychological symbiosis. They are registered at this site from the massive impingments of birth and serve as the nidus for consolidation of all aspects of bad self-experience into a whole. The dimension of biophysiological demand, with an intensity that cannot be fully contained within the nuclear self, registers an impression with the qualities of an independent object. This is represented at the interior as the bad instinctual aspect of the object and serves as the nidus for consolidating the varied impressions of a bad object's influence into an entity. The object-impression counterpart of the background object is registered at the periphery with the characteristics of a transitional object. It is the essence of a good object's influence and serves as the nidus around which the good object impressions of optimal gratification and optimal frustration consolidate to form the representation of a whole good object.

Each represented facet of experience serves a purpose and is elaborated into a fantasy that is capable of a linking function. The representation of a whole good self is composed of the following: (1) The background object of primary identification, which is elaborated into a fantasy of union with nature. This provides the experience of containment and a background for continuing mental expansion. (2) The autonomous ego functions, which are elaborated into fantasies of potential talents and skills. These provide the mental foundation for the exercise of motor and conceptual activities and establish the perceptual boundaries for the self. (3) Phase-specific instinctual gratification, which is elaborated into fantasies that expand in accordance with the nature of the instinctual experience. During the oral phase, it is of a boundless breast. As development proceeds, instinctual experience includes anal qualities of mastery and control of bodily processes, and a fantasy of omnipotence is elaborated. This incorporates libidinal activity, which functions to enable attachment to an object.

The representation of a whole good object is composed of three facets: (1) The transitional object, which is elaborated into a fantasy that establishes the mental background for transitional space. This provides the psychological space necessary for the formation of new mental structures. The linkages that will connect the two systems of reprsentation require a contained space in which they can develop. (2) The impressions of optimal frustration, which are elaborated into fantasies of mirroring. These reflect the influences of an object that have resulted in an amplification of the autonomous ego functions. The fantasy of mirroring is an image of empathic resonance, so attuned to the available functions in the self that control and regulation are attained through the use of those functions. (3) The impressions of optimal gratification, which are elaborated in fantasies consonant with the nature of the instinctual activity that is in the ascendency. During the oral phase, the fantasy is of an all-giving nurturer. In the anal phase, the impression is of an object's providing optimal opportunity for mastery, autonomy, and control, which is elaborated into a fantasy of the object's omnipotence.

The representation of a whole bad self is composed of the following: (1) The reactions to impingement, which are elaborated into fantasies of fight, flight, and withdrawal. In the earliest phases of development, these have served as a differentiating influence and continue to provide a defensive function. (2) Sensory deprivation, which is elaborated into a fantasy of emptiness. These experiences of unrealized potentials, when not excessive, lend themselves to ease the effects of overstimulation. (3) Instinctual overstimulation, which is elaborated into fantasies that correspond to the particular instinctual experience that has necessitated defense. In orality, it is of greed. As the inadequately neutralized libidinal and aggressive drives of anality are represented, the fantasy is of anal sadism.

The representation of a whole bad object is composed of the following: (1) The bad instinctual impressions, which are elaborated into primal scene fantasies. These fantasies reflect the influence of that dimension of biophysiological demand that is of an intensity that it cannot be represented. It is of an ominous, unseen, instinctual presence that is potentially traumatic. This functions as the portal of entry of instinctual demand and advances along the lines of psychosexual development. (2) The impressions of an impinging object, which are elaborated into fantasies that are shaped by the instinctual impingements. During orality, it is of an enveloping, cannibalistic object. With the emergence of anality, the impressions and associated fantasies are anally sadistic. When in proper balance, they provide a restraining and regulating influence that abets differentiation. (3) The impressions of a depriving object, which are elaborated into fantasies of withholding. Later in development, these impressions of deprivation lend themselves to being elaborated into fantasies of an idealized object. They reflect the qualities deficient in the self and sought after from an object.

When the representations of good self-experience have been sufficiently consolidated at the interior, the healing of the early splits eventuates in an alignment of consolidated entities that have evolved into systems of mental functioning. The representations of good self-experiences, which have moved to the periphery, and of bad self-experiences, which have receded into the interior, form one system. These entities maintain a connection through the line of continuity of instinctual experience. The representations of a good object's influence at the periphery and of a bad object's influence at the interior form a second system. These entities maintain a connection through the line of continuity of prohibitive experience. The varied experiences with a multitude of external objects are also being represented in the shadow of those that are primary. Fantasy elaborations stand in readiness as potential linkages for the development of new mental structures that unite and differentiate the two systems, establish self-cohesiveness, and facilitate the expression of derivatives that produce meaning.

The Formation of the First Fixation Point: The Onset of Cohesiveness

The fusion–merger experiences of a psychological symbiosis are dependent upon a lack of differentiation between self and nonself. The inability to differentiate is sustained by a quality of empathic responsiveness that does not elicit primitive, reactive defenses. The mechanism of splitting has facilitated the consolidation of the resulting good self-experiences at the interior, by enabling the reactions to inevitable impingements and deprivations to coalesce and organize at the periphery. When good self-experience is sufficiently represented and structuralized, the capacity for self-differentiation gradually becomes functional. This capacity is intially manifested in the healing of ego splits, as the ongoing representation of good self-experience moves closer to the source of empathic stimuli at the periphery. Concurrently, the ongoing representation of bad self-experience recedes to the site of instinctual impingements at the interior. The structured containing influence of good self-experience remains at the interior, and the structured differentiating influence of reactions to impingement remains at the periphery. It requires a significant degree of self-differentiation to engage in a search for the influence of a good object because the regressive pull of fusion and merger experiences is very active. The process of separation–individuation is initiated by this progressive movement toward continuing growth and self-expansion.

The representation of the experience of extending perceptual activity around the structured remnants of reactions to impingement expands the boundaries of the self. When the coalescing impressions of a good object's influence are recognized, these boundaries can include the evolving system of object representations. The search for a good object's influence has formed two arms of perception and a focused area of internal perceptual activity.

The represented extension of the self-system forms an introjective arm of perception. This functions as a perceptual pathway for stimuli to be internalized and as a foundation for introjective processes. The represented recognition of a good object's influence forms a projective arm of perception. This will function as a perceptual pathway for the influences of an object, which is the foundation for projective processes. The focused area of perceptual activity forms the eye of consciousness and has the function of self-observation.

The initial perception of a good object as separate is very unstable. The exercise of the autonomous ego functions has to operate at its fullest capacity for it to be maintained. With fatigue or stress, it is readily lost and then regained. The perception can only be stabilized with the differentiating influence of the good object's bad qualities. The line of continuity of prohibitive experience, represented as optimal frustration in the good object and shading into the impingements represented in the bad object, provides a pathway for this recognition. The object and its representations are established as separate, by the formation of this first fixation point on the projective arm of perception. In health, this occurs during the anal period and promotes further differentiation.

Concurrently, there is a continuing progression in the representation of experience that is interrelated with the effects of maturation. That which is instinctually gratifying has been changing from the oral components important for early primitive introjective processes to anal components that embody mastery and control of bodily functions. The formation of this first fixation point has transpired in conjunction with the establishment of consensual validation; that is, the perceptual processes function in concert with each other. The eye of consciousness (a psychic expression of visual perceptual experience) depends upon an integration of the representational functions evoked by the near receptors with the organizational functions evoked by the distant receptors.

The Formation of Unifying and Differentiating Structures: The Grandiose Self and Ego Ideal

The experience, associated with the recognition of the object as separate from the self, is one of helplessness and vulnerability. This motivates the need to establish a connection to the influence of an object that can balance that experience. Libidinal self-representations, which involve experiences of mastery and control during the anal period, express their binding function in seeking attachment to an object. The impression of an optimally gratifying anal object is elaborated into a fantasy of its omnipotence. This fantasy is a perfect match for alleviating the feeling of extreme vulnerability. A structured union is effected between the representations of a good instinctual self and object through a fantasy of the object's omnipotence. I have called it the ''grandiose self'' because it is based upon participation in a fantasy. This new structure functions to more effectively unite and differentiate the two systems of representation and to form the foundation for internal regulation of continuing self-expansion.

The formation of a healthy grandiose self signifies that there is trust in the reliability of external objects. Good self-experience has been sufficiently represented and structuralized at the interior to establish a foundation; it is stable enough to be weakened by participating in a fantasy. A healthy grandiose self is vital for the continuation of progressive steps in development. When there is an insufficiency of good qualities in experience, unstable and distorted differentiating linkages may form that are severely depleting and increase the state of vulnerability. The consequence is in accentuating the need for regulation through continued dependence on the external world.

The formation of the grandiose self weakens the adaptive and sublimatory functions in the self-system of representations. A motive is present to utilize the represented influences of an object to regain strength and stability. The advancing process of separation-individuation has founded a perceptual pathway to the varied representations of an object's influence, through the development of a fixation point and the evolving function of self-observation. The potential skills and functions of the self have been elaborated into fantasies that are available to serve a linking function. Those functions, which are most deficient, can then link to the representation of an object that is most needed (and hence admired). The resulting structure is based on this process of selective identification, and for that reason, I have called it the "ego ideal." It serves to further unite and differentiate the two systems of representation. In health, it is primarily the impressions of an optimally frustrating good object that are most needed and admired. However, under transient periods of stress or overstimulation, there may be a need for the restraining influence of a prohibitive bad object. When these identifications with an aggressor predominate, it is an expression of the emergence of pathology.

Two new structures have formed. One, the grandiose self, is an instinctual structure and is particularly suited to regulate primary process mental activity. In being linked to the fantasy of an object's mental impression, it is consonant with the regulatory needs of the pleasure principle. The second, the ego ideal, is a structure based on selective identifications and is particularly suited to regulate secondary process mental activity. In being linked to the mental impression of an external object's influence, it is more affected by the external world and consonant with the regulatory needs of the reality principle.

The Formation of Perceptual Boundaries within the Self: The Superego Eye

The systems of conscious, preconscious, and unconscious mental activities are delineated by the formation of perceptual boundaries. These are focused areas of perceptual activity that are particularly adapted to register psychic activity within a given realm and are in harmony with the regulatory principles that govern that realm.

The experience of recognizing the mental impressions of a separate good object's influence has expanded the perceptual boundaries of the self. The interior border is attuned to the internal world and develops a focused area of inwardly directed perceptual activity. It is consolidated and organized to function as the eye of consciousness. The exterior border is attuned to the external world and is consolidated and organized to register the immediate impressions of its stimuli. The perceptual movement around the structured remnants of reactions to impingement, necessary to locate the representation of a good object, has created a sector of transitional space. This is the psychological space within which the immediate impressions of external stimuli are registered and that will contain the symbolic productions of an evolving system of conscious mental activity.

The focuses of inwardly directed perceptual attention associated with the interior border and of outwardly directed perceptual attention associated with the exterior border are incorporated in the new structures that unite and differentiate the two systems of representation. The grandiose self is an instinctual structure designed to balance the experience of vulnerability, through participation in a fantasy of the good object's omnipotence. It forms along the perceptual pathway of inwardly directed attunement to the influence of a good object. The interior border is incorporated and develops a focused area of inwardly directed perceptual attention. The ego ideal, designed to amplify and strengthen the self through the influences of an object, is a structure based upon selective identifications. It forms along the perceptual pathway of externally directed attunement. The exterior border is incorporated, and a focused area of outwardly directed perceptual attention is developed. These perceptual functions are gradually organizing to give definition to varying systems of consciousness.

In conjunction with the formation of the grandiose self and ego ideal, a new consolidated area of perceptual functioning has been established in the realm of transition from conscious to unconscious mental activity. It parallels the perceptual activity of the eye of consciousness (directed inward) and of immediate perceptions (directed outward) that have been organized to function at the periphery. The inner border is a part of, and regulated by, the grandiose self. The outer border is a part of, and regulated by, the ego ideal. I have called this focus of perceptual activity the "superego eye" because it is a structural precursor of what will eventually become the superego. It forms the perceptual boundaries of an evolving preconscious system of mental activity.

The grandiose self is a relatively unstable structure, as it is based on the fantasy of an object's influence. Its perceptual border delineates the transition from an unconscious to a preconscious system of mental activity and must be concordant with the pleasure principle that guides the id of the dynamic unconscious. The grandiose self is not bound to external reality and is thus capable of regulating the fluid cathectic shifts and condensations necessary for the primary process to operate. The ego ideal is a stable structure, as it is based on the mental impressions of an external object's influence. Its perceptual border delineates the transition from a preconscious to a conscious system of mental activity and must be concordant with the reality principle that guides the conscious system. The ego ideal is bound to external reality and is thus capable of regulating the linear, logical, sequential thinking and immediate perceptions necessary for the secondary process to operate.

A system of conscious mental activity has evolved, which is bounded by two areas of focused perceptual functioning. One, the eye of consciousness, is directed inward from the surface of the personality. The second, the border of the ego ideal, is directed outward to the same mental contents from a more regressed perspective. The realm of preconscious mental activity has not as yet evolved into a well-defined system but is gradually organizing its boundaries. The superego eye, formed by the perceptual borders of the grandiose self and ego ideal, delineate the transitions that characterize this preconscious system. In these early narcissistic stages of development, the boundary for the unconscious system is formed by the representations of instinctual impingements and the reactions to them. This is an anxiety-laden realm, dominated by the heightened need for defensive activity. The border of the grandiose self has developed a focused area of perceptual functioning that is directed inward to register the contents of the emerging preconscious system. These contents are primarily the images of self- and object linkages that are increasingly proliferating and will function as derivatives to express unconscious mental activity.

The fixation point on the projective arm of perception provides the stability that is necessary for these structures, borders, and perceptual functions to organize. It is essential that the introjective arm of perception not be fixated at this point in development, in order to enable the ongoing representation of new experiences. The expanding representation of the component instincts facilitates progression toward a genital consolidation. A fixation point on the introjective arm of perception, based on a recognition of the good self's bad qualities, is only transiently necessary during the period of oedipal organization.

A Brief Look to the Future: The Relationship of Cohesiveness to the Oedipal Conflict

Cohesiveness is initiated when the boundaries of the self are expanded to include the representations of an object. This occurs with the recognition of a separate good object's influence and is readily lost until a fixation point is established. This perception of a good object's bad qualities has a differentiating effect that stabilizes cohesiveness but is associated with an experience of tremendous helplessness and vulnerability. The availability of an object's influence internally enables self-regulatory functions to develop, and a new structure is formed to balance the experience of vulnerability. This new structure, the grandiose self, links the representations of good instinctual self-experience to the fantasy of an optimally gratifying object's omnipotence. The effect is to more firmly secure cohesiveness and to deplete the adaptive capacities of the self. A motive is present to utilize the representations of an object so as to strengthen these adaptive functions. Another new structure, the ego ideal, links the fantasies of self-potentials to the needed and admired impressions of an object. The weakening of the self that occurred through belief in a fantasy is buttressed by a concomitant belief in a reality, and cohesiveness is anchored at the periphery. Although cohesiveness is strengthened, it cannot be continuously maintained and ensured until the genital fantasies of the oedipal conflict unite the two systems of representation at the interior.

The process of structuralizing the linkage of two functional systems of representation, so that they are both united and differentiated, requires a stabilizing influence. The fixation point on the projective arm of perception has served that purpose as the grandiose self and ego ideal were formed. With the formation of the ego ideal, perceptual attention is directed into the self-system of representations. This occurs at a time when the component instincts are organizing into a gential consolidation, in preparation for the elaboration of an oedipal conflict. These are the genital fantasies that provide the necessary linkages for new structure formation at the interior. The increase in intensity of instinctual activity necessitates a greater degree of perceptual stability during the period of oedipal organization. The recognition of the good self's bad qualities, through the line of continuity of instinctual experience, establishes a fixation point on the introjective arm of perception that fulfills that requirement. This fixation point provides the stability that enables the lines of continuity of instinctual and prohibitive experience to consolidate into the regulatory structure of castration anxiety and for the oedipal conflict to evolve without the disruptive effect of an influx of new experience. The stage is set for the organizing influence of the oedipal conflict to unite all aspects of the self and object and to insure cohesiveness in a manner that allows for a continuing self-expansion.

When cohesiveness and continuity of experience are well established in the personality, the mental impressions of an object's influence are accessible for attaining advancing degrees of self-regulation. Concurrent with the elaboration of an oedipal conflict, the differentiating structures of the grandiose self and ego ideal operate as a foundation for consolidation of the superego as an independently functioning agency. Initially, the evolving functions of the superego are manifested in separate sectors of the personality. An instinctual pathway to the system of object representations, organized at the projective arm of perception, has been established with the formation of the grandiose self. The idealizing superego functions are in evidence at this locale. The pathway of selective identification with the representations of an object has been established with the formation of the ego ideal. This is the vehicle by which the influence of an object is included within the self-system of representations that is organized at the introjective arm of perception. The prohibitive functions of the superego are in evidence at this locale, when the need for powerful restraint instigates identifications with the impinging aspect of a bad object. This identification with an aggressor is perceptually accessible through the line of continuity of prohibitive experience. The separation in function is a parallel of the earlier splits in the ego, prior to the onset of cohesiveness. The pathway of the ego ideal is also utilized for the selective identifications that lead to a resolution of the oedipal conflict and integrate the splits in the superego. The effect is to insure cohesiveness throughout the personality.

The structures that form during the course of development reflect the individual's efforts to adapt to the internal and external environments. Each structure has the potential for a healthy or pathological outcome. An exposition of their developmental lines in health provides a theoretical foundation for determining the significance of their distortion with pathology. It also aids in discerning that which is healthy and that which is pathological in a given individual.

Discussion

A's physical "attack" upon the therapist's belongings was reminiscent of his earlier behavior, in which he appeared to be admonishing his hands against reaching out to the environment. *A* was now actively engaging himself with the therapist, in what appeared to be an effort to determine the depth of the therapist's understanding. Earlier, the therapist had imposed his own inner conflicts upon *A*, and it had been devastating. An impinging environment was created, to which *A* could only adapt by reestablishing his autistic position. The qualities of good self-experience were so poorly represented in *A*'s early development that they were both fragmented and unavailable. He had disengaged himself from the traumatic effects of an unempathic environment. That disengagement was sustained by maintaining the fragmented representations of bad self-experience at the point of contact with the external world. When the therapist slowly communicated an awareness of how impinging he had been, it seemed to encourage *A* to more actively test the therapist's ability to function with the qualities of a good object. Words were not enough, and *A* had to elicit the more powerful impact of a physical interaction. In the process of doing so, he experienced his ability to be effective in reaching out to touch the external environment. *A*'s "attack" upon the therapist's belongings created an atmosphere in which the inner intent of the therapist could be experienced through physical contact. the stimulus of physical contact invokes a much more powerful body ego experience.

During these interactions, *A* offered many communicative statements that seemed to portray the manner in which the effects of biophysiological demands were represented. This was most clearly illustrated in his descriptions of the Make-A-Dos. These figures varied from having pleasurable instinctual qaualities that did not require defense, to having impinging instinctual qualities that required defense, to having ominous and frightening instinctual qualities that assumed the proportions of an independent instinctually threatening object. They appeared to reflect a line of continuity of instinctual experience that was represented as a facet of the good and bad selves and of a bad object.

The physical interaction with *A* made the effect of the therapist's containing function more visible. His increasing capacity to communicate verbally was one indication that the representations of good self-experience were consolidated into a whole. The Make-A-Dos, rather than being live internal presences that dominated *A*, came to be mental productions that reflected his internal experience. A could talk about them as memories or products of his imagination, which was in contrast to his being filled with their influence and helpless in regulating the experience. The concept of a self with object qualities was helpful in defining the original body ego experience by which a stimulus outside of the self could be included within the self.

An interrelationship became evident between the way instinctual experience was represented and the empathic qualities that were present in the interaction. When the therapist provided a consistent experience of empathic responsiveness and containment, the Make-A-Dos were fun loving, did not require defense, and were represented as a facet of good self-experience. When the therapist's empathic responsiveness was consistent and uninterrupted over long stretches of time, A became immersed in an internal state in which the distinctions between self-experience and the impressions of an object were blurred. This period of lack of differentiation was interrupted by the frustration introduced with a change in the therapist's attitude. A's response to the frustration indicated that a more firmly consolidated self-experience was available to him. It appeared that, during the period of a lack of differentiation, a stimulus outside of the self (the interaction with the empathically responding therapist) had been included within the self (a firmer representation of a whole good self and the representation of the new figure of the soldier). The effect was to amplify and expand upon the containing function of the background object of primary identification. The concepts of the object with self-qualities and the self with object qualities seemed to offer a construct to explain the manner in which new representational structures are formed.

The devastating effect of the therapist's empathic lapse indicated the fragility of these new representational structures. When the therapist rectified his attitude, however, they could reassert their presence. A initiated physical contact in an attempt to verify the therapist's capacity for empathic responsiveness. He designed a stiuation in which he could be perceived as expressing hostility when he was reaching out for comfort and containment. This recreated the scenario of the earlier impingement and was probably a reflection of his original developmental traumata. A gradually began to communicate with the therapist, and in doing so, gave evidence of being accessible to the therapeutic interaction. It was an indication that the representations of good self-experience had coalesced into a whole and had risen to the surface (the point of perceptual contact with the external world). The representations of bad self-experience appeared to have receded into the interior, leaving a readiness to respond defensively at the surface. It was at this point that A exhibited the capacity to recognize the separateness of the therapist as a good object and, by implication, the representation of the experience.

This recognition of the separateness of a good object was associated with an experience of vulnerability and helplessness. It was the first time that such a feeling state was clearly evident in his communications and in his behavior. At the same time, communicative descriptions of interactions with a variety of external objects were emerging as a new development. The particular nature of these communications expressed his efforts to attain mastery and control, which reflected the budding ability to link representations of the self and object to form instinctual derivatives. Anal qualities of good self-experience had become predominant, indicative of his expanding capcity for instinctual representation.

A's response to the feeling of vulnerability was to search for a way to gain a sense of balance. A new structure was formed by linking the instinctual qualities of mastery and control to the omnipotent fantasy of a good optimally gratifying object. The fantasy of A as a special agent, gaining increasing mastery of his environment, and the therapist, as the head of the special agents, reflected the emergence of this new structure. I have called it the "grandiose self." A's great delight in participating in the fantasy offered a sense of balance to his profound feeling of vulnerability. However, his ability to exercise adaptive functions was weakened until he became visibly more introspective. As A adopted the qualities of introspection, previously attributed to the therapist, he became more effective in his ability to adapt and attain mastery in the various areas of his functioning.

Another new structure was formed when A was able to elaborate his own potentials into fantasies that were then linked to the introspective qualities of the therapist that he needed and admired. I have called this structure the "ego ideal" because it was created by a process of selective identification. The self-representational system was depleted by participating in a fantasy of the object's omnipotence and was bolstered by including qualities of an object that strengthened the exercise of its functions.

When A was confronted with a physical separation from the therapist, profound anxiety emerged due to the tenuous organization of these newly formed structures. A was fearful that his ability to sustain self-regulation would be disrupted when he was not in actual contact with the therapist. This was expressed in his concern that the airplane would crash or not get off of the ground. His anxiety also resonated with the previous trauma that had occurred following a physical separation. At this time A had been in a similarly vulnerable position. The trauma had occurred as a result of an empathic failure by the therapist, not as a result of the separation. The therapist's interpretation that A was concerned about his capacity to maintain the image of the therapist seemed to strengthen the function of these newly formed structures (the grandiose self and ego ideal). It also evoked an image symbolic of the previous trauma, which was expressed in his anxiety concerning the return trip. He found a way to maintain mastery of the impending separation but could feel his dependence upon the therapist. The therapist's recognition of this anxiety had the effect of more firmly solidifying the continuity of these differentiating structures. This was most clearly communicated by his telephone call. A was reporting to the therapist that he felt safe in being separate. The telephone call also manifested his need to receive further amplification through this contact.

This new development was associated with an increasing capacity to form, perceive, and communicate derivatives. The concept that the structures of the grandiose self and ego ideal develop focused areas of perceptual activity was useful in explaining the emergence of this new perceptual function. Derivatives formed by linking representations of the self and object could now be perceived and communicated. The process of uniting and differentiating the two systems of representation, the establishment of cohesiveness, the capacity for production of meaning, and the mechanism of derivative formation were all interrelated and interdependent developments. In an earlier, primitive level of psychic organization, A was able to communicate derivatives, but they were reactive in nature, fragmented, and dependent upon the therapist's capacity to construct and infer their meaning, rather than being an expression of the presence of meaning.

F was a child whose pathology interfered with the communication of meaning, although he had developed consolidated representations of a whole good and bad self and established a cohesive attachment to the representations of an object. His entire manner of adapting to the therapeutic interaction was based upon idealizations. Idealizations are an attempt to compensate for deficiencies in the self-representational system, by elaborating fantasies of their presence in the influence of an object. The depriving object is thereby perceived as having the qualities missing in the self. The effect is to further weaken and deplete the self-representational system and to debilitate adaptive functioning. Rather than participating in the object's omnipotence, to balance the vulnerability of separateness, effort must be exerted to create it. In addition, idealizations interfere with the process of selective identification and establish cohesiveness upon the debilitating effects of compensatory efforts. The consequence was best described by F in his portrayal of the therapeutic interaction. He felt as though there were two of him—one in the forefront, talking, and one in the background, watching the therapist. The foreground figure idealized the therapist. The background figure was weak and ineffective. This description fits what Winnicott (1958) has referred to as the false and true selves.

In the early months, F derivatively expressed the feeling of hiding from, deceiving, and fooling the therapist. The therapist recognized the significance of these derivative expressions but was unable to communicate his awareness effectively. The therapist's ability to interpret was affected by the absence of a context that could give unity to F's productions. There was always a missing ingredient in these derivative expressions, either the representation of an object, of the self, or the fantasy linkage. This was partly a result of defensive activity in F, designed to maintain this facade, and partly a function of the therapist's mode of participation. The therapist's assumption that F's mental activities had meaning was an obstacle to understanding the interaction. The therapist, in confusion and frustration, offered linear interpretations that directed attention to the conscious system. The quality of the ensuing interaction illustrates the debilitating effects of these interpretations. The therapist unwittingly reinforced an ongoing process of destruction of meaning, by directing attention to the conscious elements of F's communications. The therapist's interpretations of F's anger, envy, and sexual anxiety reinforced his defensive posture and interfered with the creation of meaning in the interaction.

A potential key to understanding the interaction was manifested in F's idealization of the therapist. This expressed his attempt to compensate for that which was missing within himself. However, it was not until the therapist grasped the significance of F's statement, "I see what you mean," that a context was available that contained in it an unconscious communication. It acquainted the therapist with the realization that he had been participating in an interaction that reinforced the destruction of meaning. It also offered the therapist a vehicle by which he could communicate his understanding. The therapist's interpretation established a connection to F that made the emergence of meaning possible.

F heard the sound of his own voice, which reflected his perception of a consolidated self united with, and differentiated from, the influence of an object. He could then also perceive the mental contents of his preconscious system, without the profound interference from defensive activities that destroyed meaning. The therapist, in establishing a communicative interaction by which meaning could be restored, was creating an environment in which pathological forces could be identified. Derivative expressions, with meaning, could now be communicated. F's recall of the story of the prince, cursed to live in a state of ugliness until he was recognized, gave validity to his feeling of being unconsciously understood. The story reflected a reactive, derivative recognition of his ugliness, which was a consequence of his distorted perception of himself. The experience of being unconsciously understood is a process of recognition and enabled a pathway toward undoing the distortions. The production of meaning makes it possible for the therapeutic interaction to influence the dissolution of pathological defenses and provide the wherewithal for integration to occur.

The mental representation of body ego experiences and object impressions and their fantasy elaborations that serve as linkages provide the framework for producing and expressing the meaning of any given human experience. A process or interaction that destroys or interferes with any one of these mental productions destroys or interferes with meaning. The task of a therapist is to conduct an interaction with a set of conditions in which meaning can take place or in which a diagnosis can be made as to what has interfered with the development of, or expression of, meaning. Conceptualizing a developmental line for the emergence of meaning can illuminate the qualities in an interaction that foster or inhibit its expression. For example, a dream, by its composition, is expressive of meaning. The background object of primary identification has provided the mental stage upon which the dream is enacted. The dream is composed of representations of body ego experiences (which are symbolized), object impressions (the objects in the dream), and fantasy linkages (the experience of the dreamer). The manner in which a dream is communicated, and the ensuing interaction, may either reinforce a process of destruction of meaning that is ongoing in the dreamer or enhance the emergence of meaning that the act of dreaming reflects.

CHAPTER 6

The Pregenital Phàses of Psychosexual Development

The Evolution of Focused Perceptual Functions and Boundaries and the Preconditions for the Establishment of an Oedipal Conflict

Introduction

The expression that "it all depends on how you look at it" captures the universal observation that a given stimulus can be perceived in different ways depending upon the attitude of the observer. It also embodies the idea that a given stimulus can be perceived in different ways simultaneously. How does this complicated act of perception take place? What is at the foundation of a capacity to perceive a differing stimulus and simultaneously the same stimulus in differing ways? The continuity of conscious to preconscious to unconscious mental activity is also dependent upon an act of perception that is occurring with differing qualities in differing sectors of the personality. It is thus important to define a developmental line of perceptual functioning that can trace the evolution of these complicated perceptual tasks.

In this presentation, a definition of the self has been determined by the activity of perception. I have been portraying the interrelationship between perception and the representational

145

functions that it activates and that, in turn, influence the ongoing process of perception. A theoretical construct has been formulated for delineating the effects of interactions with external objects and the means by which the stimuli of the internal world of biophysiological demand are registered. Body ego experiences, evoked by the activity of perception, are registered to form the system of self-representations. The manner in which stimuli affect perceptual processes are registered as object impressions and develop into a system of object representations. These mental representations are then available to expand the capacity for registering the impact of biophysiological demand. A metapsychology that is based upon this interdependent interrelationship allows for a fuller integration of self-psychology, object relations theory, and instinctual theory. The integration is determined by the effects of perception and adds an ego psychological point of view.

The effects upon mental processes of empathic lapses and failures is especially noteworthy. They tend to highlight the differing qualities of perception in various sectors of the personality. The perception of an empathic failure is expressed one way in the conscious system and in quite another way in the preconscious and unconscious systems. These empathic lapses and failures are often the fulcrums around which a therapeutic interaction revolves. It is sometimes stated, either explicitly or implicitly, that a therapeutic process depends upon the presence of some minimal degree of empathic failure. Yet, when empathic responsiveness is consistently present, the therapeutic process flows with continuity and effectiveness. The nature of psychological disturbances is such that, given a containing, trustable, and nonimpinging interaction, increasing degrees of disturbed inner psychic contents enter the realm of conscious experience. The intensity of these psychological forces, when expressed in an interaction, often evokes the defensive responses of both parties. The patient's task is to bring these pathological forces into the interaction. The therapist's task is to monitor the various reactions to them, undo the defensive aspects, and offer an interpretation of the unconscious meaning of the communication. I have often wondered how it is that an empathic lapse or failure can be an impetus to one patient and foster further and deeper therapeutic work, whereas for another patient, or even the same patient on another occasion, it can serve as an obstacle to therapeutic progress.

In every case, it was essential that the therapist's failure in empathy was rectified before progress could occur. Some patients seemed to have much tolerance as that process of rectification took place. Most patients were active participants in discovering the source of an empathic failure, usually in the form of expressing derivatives of unconscious perceptions. There were other situations in which an empathic failure was not tolerated or even created a dissolution of the therapeutic experience. The reasons were many and varied. They depended upon the depth and seriousness of the failure, the particular meaning to the patient, and the degree of flexibility within the therapist. However, an additional consideration appeared to be a significant factor. This involved the patient's capacity to contain the effects of the lapse and to communicate the derivative associations that potentially might guide the therapist; that is, to function as a supervisor to the therapist.

The ability to tolerate empathic failures, and to participate in their rectification, has seemed to depend upon the patient's capacity to maintain an intrapsychic connection to the representation of an object. Although any psychic content can be viewed as reflecting the impact of the therapeutic interaction, these unions serve a regulatory function and provide the wherewithal to communicate the individual meaning of a given interaction. The degree of success in negotiating separation–individuation was in direct proportion to the presence of represented attachments of the self and object. The developmental step of uniting and differentiating these two systems of representation resulted in an increasing ability to integrate greater degrees of instinctual demand. New ways of perceiving inner and outer worlds emerged, and derivatives of instinctual activity and unconscious perceptions could be formed to communicate individual meaning more effectively.

The shift from oral to anal aspects of instinctual representation is also a shift from the incorporative position of taking things in, to the position of attaining mastery and control. Aggressive instinctual activity, when well contained and regulated, has the effect of fostering differentiation and motivating assertiveness. It is essential for experiences of mastery and control to be viable. When aggression is poorly regulated, it is destructive to mental structuralization. This is a particularly crucial matter in individuals whose early development has been dominated by overwhelming amounts of aggression and in whom there is little available to contain or regulate it. In working with such individuals, I have been impressed by its seeming total absence until a therapeutic symbiosis was experienced. It was only in emerging from this undifferentiated state that aggression could be contained and represented within the self. In addition to the appearance of aggression, communication shifted from depending upon the therapist to infer meaning to being able to communicate with meaning.

The increased ability to communicate meaning was associated with an advance in instinctual representation. Anal experiences of mastery and control gradually shifted to phallic experiences with exhibitionistic qualities. The autistic children I worked with, who were able to negotiate the process of separation–individuation, each entered a phase of phallic exhibitionism that acquainted me with its healthy aspects. It emerged as a phallic instinctual activity that did not require defense and was represented as a facet of good self-experience. However, it was often poorly regulated and rapidly developed an intensity that was accompanied by anxiety and required a defensive response. At this stage, there was a profound difference in the way anxiety affected psychological functioning. Previously, anxiety had been crippling and debilitating, indicated the failure of a regulatory function, and manifested a threat to the integrity of the self. Now anxiety functioned to signal a defensive response. An effective, underlying structure appeared to have developed as a foundation for anxiety that reflected a new level of psychic organization. It appeared to me, that for this signaling function of anxiety to be present, the underlying structure must have linkages to all aspects represented in the self and object. This degree of organization only transpired when instinctual expansion had reached phallic and genital levels of experience. The anxiety of castration was the only manifestation of anxiety that served a signaling function.

Negotiating the separation–individuation phase has involved a consolidation of body ego experiences into a system of self-representations, and the structuralization of fantasy linkages to unite and differentiate the two systems. Perceptual functions are incorporated in these new mental structures to enable the gradual evolution of the differing qualities of perception that give definition to a conscious, preconscious, and unconscious system of mental activity. Each area of focused perceptual activity is on a line of continuity to the other, and a given stimulus is exposed to these differing qualities of perception simultaneously.

In this chapter, I will describe the pregenital phases of psychosexual development and delineate the varied experiences that are represented as facets of the self and object. Their particular fantasies will be highlighted because they reflect the composition of underlying unions and mental structures. The evolution of focused areas of perceptual activity throughout the personality and the emergence of a conscious, preconscious, and unconscious system of mental activity will be discussed further. The discussion will include the makeup of the differing perceptual boundaries and their relationship to the principles that govern each system. I will also reexamine the formation and function of fixation points in relation to the structure of castration anxiety. Finally, I will review and emphasize the early developmental events that must be negotiated for the establishment of an oedipal conflict.

Clinical Material

A returned from his trip filled with descriptions of his activities and reactions. In this way, he indicated that he was continuing where he had left off. He felt confidence in himself and in the therapist. In the ensuing months, at first gradually and then with increasing regularity, *A* began to be absorbed with a feeling of anger and an enormous fear of asserting himself. He would begin slowly and, as he talked, became increasingly angry. His body movements became stiff and rigid, and he appeared very frightened. It looked as though he could barely contain the intensity of his inner experience. In vivid terms, he emphasized how much he wanted to be angry and not hold himself back. He described interactions in which he had felt put down, controlled, or forced into submission. This enraged him and stimulated fantasies of extreme violence. He began to talk of his admiration for General Patton. He was a hero, and *A* wished he could be just like him. The therapist reflected on *A*'s wish to find these qualities in the therapist and to include them as a part of himself. *A* immediately stated that he had made a decision. He had enough, was no longer going to be submissive, and was firmly determined to no longer hold back in expressing his anger. Immediately following that assertion, he developed an explosive diarrhea. The diarrhea lasted several weeks and became severe enough to raise concerns about dehydration.

During this time, *A* expressed the idea that his body was speaking for him. His decision to express aggression flooded him with an intensity that was uncontainable. The diarrhea subsided, and, as it did, *A* began to laugh. He thought of himself being filled with anger and spilling it out in his diarrhea. He continued to talk about his rage. He paced back and forth, shaking his hand and head as he did. His whole being vibrated. His mannerisms were again reminiscent of that period of time when he appeared to be berating and admonishing his hands. This behavior was now associated with verbalizations of intense aggression. He stated that he felt like a bomb ready to explode.

A began to direct his fury at his mother and erupted when she made any demand. Her response was of repulsion accompanied by a whiny appeal, "Oh, *A*, why do you have to be this way?" *A* then was overcome with a feeling of his badness. He found it impossible to be openly angry with his father, because he felt frightened and paralyzed. He continued to exert an effort to stand up for himself and express his anger. When he did, it came out with such force that people looked at him as though he were crazy. The slightest demand or question elicited a very angry and shouted "Why!" that was followed by a profound sense of humiliation.

The therapist occasionally commented on *A*'s concern that he would be injured by *A*'s attacks or that *A*'s anger would ignite a similar feeling in the therapist. *A*'s immediate reaction to even the first word uttered by the therapist was an angrily shouted "Why! did you say that!" The therapist reflected back upon *A*'s associations, and he would then state, "Oh, I see." He went on to say that he felt like he was practicing to be angry with the therapist and test his ability to be openly angry. He did not feel crazy or humiliated, and he could react without feeling bad.

Slowly *A* became more contained and comfortable with his aggression and even spoke of the pleasure it gave him to be assertive. This instituted a shift to *A*'s preoccupation with genital sensations. He talked of masturbatory activities and of his wish to rub his penis in the sessions. The therapist interpreted the wish as reflecting *A*'s experience of sexual fantasies that he wanted to talk about in therapy. The following session occurred immediately afterward.

A entered quietly with a determined look on his face. He was struggling with an internal decision. He finally shook his head affirmatively, took out his penis, and began to rub it. The therapist stated that *A* must have heard his words as an invitation to masturbate. *A* spoke of his pleasure in masturbating and said that it seemed to make the therapist uncomfortable when he did. *A*'s ability to assert himself made the therapist aware of his discomfort in being a participant in this sexual experience. The therapist reflected upon the accuracy of *A*'s perception. *A* was delighted and continued to exhibit his erect penis. He remembered a time when he worried whenever his penis got erect. He was afraid it would break or that it was defective. The therapist commented that his uneasiness in watching had seemed to remind *A* of his own previous concern. *A* continued to masturbate in silence and then recalled a dream he had the previous evening. He and a man were construction workers. They were building a very high, new, strong concrete building. The building was unfinished, and they were working on the thirteenth floor. Looking down, he could see the remnants of an old rundown shack that had been removed to construct the new building. He recalled looking to see how high the building was to be but was unable to see the top.

G was a 31-year-old man who sought therapeutic help for what he initially described as occasional episodes of impotence. It later emerged that *G* had suffered from ejaculatory impotence his entire life. His sense of shame and humiliation was so extreme that he could hardly bear to admit it to himself. He began psychoanalytic therapy four sessions per week, and this quality of extreme shame and humiliation dominated the early months. He worked hard to present himself as a happy, well-adjusted, easygoing person who was capable of managing any difficulty and who only periodically had minor disturbances. At the same time that he was presenting himself in this fashion, derivative associations reflected the severity of his trouble. During this period, he dreamt of being on a boat, ready to take a long ocean voyage, and noticed the boat was rocking horribly. He was anxious as to whether the boat could stay afloat and noticed that it had not yet left the harbor.

It took many months for G to slowly become aware of the extent of his denial and of the depth of his shame and humiliation. During this time, the therapist's silence was experienced as intensely frustrating. These experiences of frustration were the means by which he gradually began to discover his inner world of feelings. For example, on one occasion he discovered a magazine in the waiting room with another person's name on it. He demanded to know why and would cry out in rage that he had a right to know: he was entitled. He was surprised at the intensity of his feeling and began to sense there was more to it than the surface meaning he clung to. He gradually came to be aware of his intense feeling of jealousy and of his struggle to deny its existence. Therapeutic inteventions, which reflected on his deep concern that the therapist would not hear the extent of his inner conflicts and would join with him in the denial of them, were extremely facilitating. Derivative responses reflected a feeling of being understood and led to a gradual revelation of the contents of his inner world.

G was the oldest of four children who experienced a very special relationship with his mother during his early years. The specialness was founded on a hidden, unspoken mutually gratifying sexual interaction. It was this quality that he constantly sought with the therapist. The relationship was interrupted by the birth of his siblings. He slowly became aware of the genital overstimulation that was present when he felt frustration with the therapist's silence. He was crying out for the therapist to talk because the therapist's words made him feel soothed and caressed. The following occurred immediately after a session in which G had described a dream that portrayed a woman's sucking on his penis. He associated the dream to his feeling about the therapist's words and to historical material concerning his mother's physical seductive care of him as a young child.

G entered the hour carrying an umbrella. It was raining, and the umbrella was wet. He asked if he could put it in a closet in the therapist's office. The door to the closet was closed. He did not want to leak water all over the therapist's office; perhaps the closet would be a good place for it. He felt that it was also a forbidden place but could feel an intense urge to put it there. The more he thought about it, the more frightened he felt. "Would it be OK?" The therapist stated that G was asking whether the therapist would participate with G in putting a part of himself into a closed and hidden place that belonged to the therapist. G lay on the couch holding his umbrella and thought of an incident when he was 5 years of age. There was excitement in the house as everyone was awaiting the arrival of a man. When he arrived, G asked who the man was and why he was there. He was told by his father that the man was a barber and that he had come to give a haircut to his new infant brother. G was puzzled and asked why his brother needed a haircut because he had so little hair, whereas he, G, had so much more. He felt totally humiliated by the laughter of the group that surrounded him. He realized later that the event was the circumcision of his younger brother. He recalled everyone disappearing into a closed room and that he could not enter. He felt terrified. He then was flooded with memories of his mother at varying periods during his childhood. She placed herself in provocative positions so that her genitals were exposed to him. He remembers being acutely aware of her and of being excited and frightened. It made him think of his lifelong feeling that it was safe and even more desirable to masturbate. He could always reach an organism that way, whereas he had never been orgastic with a woman. Sexual encounters were always attractive and frightening, and he had developed the ability to mask his ejaculatory impotence. As the session ended, G looked up and reflected that, although the therapist had said very little, he had a feeling the therapist had talked a lot. Following the session, G had his first experience of potency in a sexual encounter.

H, an 8-year-old girl, entered therapy following her mother's contact with school. She daydreamed and ignored any situation that demanded effort and concentration. The school had done psychological testing, and the examiner had commented that this was the most deprived child she had ever seen. This was a shock to the mother who felt she had provided H with everything she needed. H was immediately eager to come to her sessions and to express her inner trouble. She felt constantly frustrated, bored, and suffered from what she called "growing pains." She felt pains in her body everywhere, which felt like something was trapped and trying to grow. The pain came from the opposition to it.

In the early months, she had many and varied pains in her ankles, fingers, stomach, and so forth. She became extremely irritable and upset with the therapist. She had the powerful sense that the therapist did not believe her and was laughing at her. Furthermore, it made no difference what the therapist would say or do or how he would respond. She just knew this was how he felt, nothing could alter that feeling, and it was terribly upsetting to her. The therapist responded that, in a way, H was right; he did not believe her. In addition, the therapist felt that H did not believe the therapist would be able to hear the way in which her body was talking to her. She seemed to fear that the therapist could not read her body's language, and she would therefore remain trapped. H's response was to talk about exploring caves, forests, bushes, and jungles. She became filled with fantasies of the thrill and danger in these explorations. The therapist said he thought her mind was occupied with exploring these spaces because she wanted the therapist to help her talk about exploring her body and its inner parts. H immediately lay on the couch and began to masturbate. She talked softly about the therapist's words giving her permission to do what she had wanted to do ever since she began to see him. She felt blocked in talking and had always known that the only way she could talk was to masturbate. The experience of rubbing herself removed the blocks, and her words came easily. She talked about a young, wild cousin and their sexual exploratory games. She recalled having seen a guard at a toll booth who frightened her and who reminded her of this cousin. She spoke of her overinvolvement with her mother. She wanted to be free of her, yet felt she could not survive without her. Her mother and father were divorced when she was 2, and H had periodic visits with her father that were both exciting and frightening. When she was with her father, she felt pulled to return to her mother. When she was back with her mother, she experienced the excited attraction to return to her father.

The Self-System of Representation in the Pregenital Phases of Psychosexual Development

The Whole Good Self

The representation of good self-experience is composed of three facets that are sufficiently disparate to be represented separately. These are qualities of experience that do not require defense and that are then integrated into an entity. They include (1) phase-specific instinctual gratification, (2) the exercise of autonomous ego functions, and (3) the background object of primary identification.

The initial instinctual experiences center around nurturing and orality, as the maternal function of containing and metabolizing the infant's reactions and responses is at its height in importance. These body ego experiences of orally phase-specific gratification are represented and elaborated into fantasies of an all-gratified, all-contained, nonfrustrated state. Instinctual advancement into the anal phase is initiated, as body ego experiences of regulation, mastery, and sphincter control rise into the ascendency. These are represented as phase-specific anal gratifications and are elaborated into fantasies of omnipotent mastery and control. The component instincts continue their growth and development to include the representations of phallic body ego experiences. This is a manifestation of an increased ability to represent greater dimensions of biophysiologic demand. It occurs in conjunction with the effects of maturation, perceptual contacts with the external world, and the formation of linkages to the representations of an object that create a richer internal world of meaning and symbolization. Body ego experiences of phallic exhibitionism are represented and are elaborated into fantasies of talents and skills being enhanced in their exhibition to an audience. There is a shift in the continuum of the self with object qualities as the demands of biophysiology are increasingly registered and greater quantities are incorporated within the realm of good self-experience. Phase-specific instinctual gratifications, represented in the good self, have expanded as a manifestation of the pregenital phases of psychosexual development (oral, anal, and phallic).

The representations of the activity of the autonomous ego functions continue to expand through the effects of maturation and through amplification, as a result of increasingly complex interactions with the object with self-qualities. Fantasies of the self's potentials are elaborated that are necessary for the process of selective identification and that serve as a foundation for the capacity to utilize thinking as trial action.

The empathic responses of the nurturing environment strengthen the stability of the background object of primary identification. This representation of the experience of containment is elaborated into fantasies of a union with mother nature. It is at the foundation of the feelings associated with perceptual contact with elements of the external natural world.

The Whole Bad Self

The representation of bad self-experience is composed of three facets that are sufficiently disparate to be represented separately. These are qualities of experience that necessitate or include a defensive response, which are then integrated into an entity. They include (1) instinctual overstimulation, (2) reactions to impingement, and (3) sensory deprivation.

The experience of instinctual overstimulation expands along the pregenital phases of psychosexual development and involves oral, anal, and phallic components. These are the body ego experiences of perceptual contact with the continuum of biophysiologic demands that are capable of representation with the aid of defense. The oral experience of instinctual overstimulation is represented as envy and greed. The fantasy elaborations are cannibalistic. As anally determined body ego experiences predominate, the overstimulating dimensions are represented as sadistic. This reflects the inadequately neutralized fusion of the libidinal and aggressive drives. They are elaborated into anally sadistic fantasies. Phallic elements of instinctual overstimulation are represented as voyeuristic. The fantasy elaborations are of forbidden, potentially humiliating, voyeuristic activities.

With advances in development, the reactions to impingement expand from primitive, reflexive responses of withdrawal to become more varied and multidimensional. When in proper proportion, these reactions are represented and serve as a foundation for the experiences of separateness and differentiation. They also operate to establish defensive activity on a firmer basis and increase the capacity to protect against overstimulation. The fantasy elaborations are of fight, flight, and withdrawal.

The body ego experience of sensory deprivation is the result of inevitable failures in empathic responsiveness and of the impossibility in providing sensory stimulation of all modalities simultaneously. The representation of these experiences reflects the effects of unrealized potentials and is elaborated into a fantasy of emptiness. The fantasy of emptiness serves well as a link to form the defensive structures necessary for the functioning of repression proper. These structures are particularly suitable when it is necessary to direct perceptual attention away from experiences that are overstimulating.

The Object System of Representations in the Pregenital Phases of Psychosexual Development

The Whole Good Object

The mental impressions of an object, possessing qualities that do not require defense, are composed of three facets sufficiently disparate to be represented separately. These are the object-impression counterparts of good self-experience, which are consolidated into the representation of a whole good object. They include the qualities of (1) optimal gratificaiton, (2) optimal frustration, and (3) a transitional object.

Optimal gratification is the instinctual aspect of a good object and reflects the influence of perceptual contact with the empathic dimension of the object with self-qualities. Initially, it is represented as a gratifying, nurturing, oral, maternal figure. A fantasy of an all-giving mother is elaborated. During the anal phase, as the conditions of optimal gratification change, it is represented as an object offering optimal opportunities for mastery and the expression of autonomy. The fantasy elaboration is of omnipotence. This representation of a good instinctual object's influence expands, during the pregenital phases of psychosexual development, to include phallic qualities. These are qualities that reflect a pleasurable response to phallic exhibitionism. It is elaborated into the fantasy of an all-admiring audience. The seeds of genital expansion begin to evolve and will be described with the lucidation of the oedipal configuration.

Optimal frustration reflects the influence of a good object's providing empathically responsive restraint in the expression of oral, anal, and phallic instinctual activities. It is the representation of an object's offering specifically those restraints that amplify dormant potentials in the self, which then become available for the exercise of regulation and control. The fantasy elaboration is of an object that perfectly mirrors functioning within the self.

The representation of a *transitional object* is the counterpart of the containing, metabolizing functions of the intrauterine environment. It has served as the original nidus of a good object's influence and expands to provide the mental foundation necessary for a stable system of object representations. The fantasy elaboration creates the transitional space within which the contents of a preconscious system are contained.

The Whole Bad Object

The mental impressions of an object, possessing qualities that require or include a defensive response, are composed of three facets sufficiently disparate to be represented separately. These are the object-impression counterparts of a bad self-experience, which are consolidated into the representaiton of a whole bad object. They include the qualities of (1) an instinctually seductive, overstimulating object; (2) an unempathic, impinging object; and (3) a depriving object.

That aspect on the continuum of biophysiologic demand with an intensity that cannot be represented within the self, even with the aid of defense, leaves a mental impression with the independent qualities of an instinctually overstimulating object. This serves as a nidus, at the interior, around which the varied impressions of a bad object's influence consolidate. It is represented in advancing oral, anal, phallic, and, later, genital dimensions. The fantasy elaborations are best characterized by the imagery of the primal scene, which can encompass the particular instinctual activity that is in the ascendency. Primal scene fantasies are of an unseen, hidden, mysterious, and ominous presence. They have the qualities of an object that is shadowy and poorly delineated, with threatening instinctual meaning. It is the experience of perceptual contact with the self with object qualities that is the source of primal scene fantasies, rather than the hidden sexual activities of an external object.

The mental impressions of an unempathic, impinging, external object are represented and affected by the instinctual impingements at the interior. Their fantasy elaborations are shaped by the particular phases of psychosexual development as they evolve. The oral fantasy is cannibalistic and devouring; the anal is sadistic, and the phallic is humiliating. A genital castrating fantasy emerges in conjunction with the consolidation of the component instincts into a genital drive that occurs later in development.

The mental impressions of a depriving object are determined by the advancing and changing conditions that are necessary for continuing self-expansion. The fantasy elaboration is of a teasing or withholding object, possessing those qualities that are most needed.

The Influence of Varied Objects

Throughout the course of development, body ego experiences and object impressions of perceptual contact with varied objects in the external world have also been represented. The most powerful experiences have centered around interactions with the primary nurturing external object. A continuum of stimuli, ranging from the most empathic to those that are unempathic and impinging, has been described as the object with self-qualities. Concurrently, the influence of varied objects has been represented in the shadow of the primary object. Initially, these are not well differentiated from the primary object, although they are reactively separate. An unfamiliar external object does not evoke the familiar representations of experience that have resulted from contact with the object with self-qualities. However, similar facets of good and bad self-experiences, their object-impression counterparts, and fantasy elaborations are represented.

With advances in perceptual maturation and the negotiation of separation–individuation, there is a clearer discrimination of the representations of varied objects. The recognition of a good object's bad qualities has stabilized self-differentiation and enhanced the capacity to discriminate the influence of varied objects. Nuances, complexities, and deepening of meaning become more viable, as these mental representations and their fantasy elaborations are available to form the derivative images that register and express psychological experience. The mechanisms of displacement, condensation, and symbolization depends upon a multiplicity of representations for their functioning.

Increasing dimensions of instinctual demand are included within self-experience as the perceptual boundaries expand, new differentiating mental structures are formed, autonomous ego functions mature, transitional space is created, and the ability to maintain memories of perceptual experience is secured. The differentiation of the differing influences of a variety of objects enables the emerging ability to be selective. A widening range of interactions become available for discovering the qualities of experience that are uniquely necessary to strengthen and stabilize adaptive capacities and that aid in achieving mastery, autonomy, and self-regulation.

The Original Transitional Object and the Creation of Transitional Space

A *transitional object* is an object in the external world that has qualities of its own, that can be shaped to be given personal meaning, and is evocative of a good object's influence. It becomes a significant element, at that specific point in development when the process of separation–individuation is asserting its presence. The effects of a transitional object indicate the existence of a mental representational counterpart that functions in the internal world. It is thus important to conceptualize the original experience with which it resonates and to determine the place it occupies in the schema of developmental progression.

In the most primitive stages of development, perceptual contact with the maternal environment *in utero* is registered in a poorly differentiated state as a bridge from the self to the nonself. The body ego experience is represented as the background object of primary identification. The object impression has all of the characteristics of a transitional object and serves as a nidus around which all of the influences of a good object will eventually coalesce. It also is the nuclear foundation upon which the influences of an object that are separate from the self can be registered, represented, and organized into a system. It is the registered experience of perceptual contact with the intrauterine environment, available at birth to be amplified by the empathic responsiveness of an external object, that establishes a psychological symbiosis. Within that symbiosis, sufficient quantities of good self-experience and a balanced proportion of bad self-experience enables the evolution of two functional systems of representation. The self-system, based on body ego experiences, consolidates at one pole. The object system, based on object impressions, consolidates with less definition at another pole. The perceptual boundaries, containing these two evolving systems, expand as an integral part of the process of separation–individuation.

Separation–individuation is concerned with attaining the recognition of a separate good object's influence. The representation of a whole good self is organized at the periphery, along with the structured remnants of reactions to impingement, as a manifestation of the healing of early splits in the ego. At the opposite pole, but also at the periphery, the mental impressions of a good object are coalescing. The original representation of a transitional object reflected the experience of a bridge between the self and the nonself. In this more differentiated state, it is the nidus of a good object's influence and is accessible to be perceived as a bridge between the separate representations of a good self and good object. Initially, the location of this bridge requires an active search that must move around the reactions to impingment. The use of this autonomous ego function and the differentiating effects of defensive reactions aid in maintaining a separation from the body ego experiences of fusion and merger.

The initial perceptual recognition of the separateness of the self and object is alternately established and lost, expanded and retracted. It remains in this unstable state until a fixation point is structured, by the recognition of the good object's bad qualities (the line of continuity of prohibitive experience). The boundaries of the self have expanded to form the eye of consciousness, an introjective and projective arm of perception, and to create a sector of psychological space. I have referred to it as "transitonal space" because it is created by extending an aspect of self-experience (the activity of perception) to an aspect of an object's influence (the representation of a transitional object). This sector of psychological space is affected by the representation of a containing experience with the external world and is thus well suited to anchor the contents of an evolving system of consciousness.

The expanded boundaries of the self have an inner and outer border that develop focused areas of perceptual activity. The inner border is perceptually attuned to look inward, reflecting the search for a good object's influence, and evolves into the eye of consciousness. The outer border is perceptually attuned to look outward, reflecting the effect of reactions to the impingements of the external world. The consolidation of the self- and object systems of representation is associated with an integration of perceptual processes into a functional unit. Consensual validation is thereby available, and the visual modality possesses the most advanced capacity for the organization of stimuli. The borders elicit the unique, characteristic reactions to a given stimulus, which the focused areas of perception register from a visual perspective.

The transitional space, created by expanding the boundaries of the self, is the psychological background for the retention of memories and immediate perceptions. There is space to anchor mental contents, boundaries to contain them, and the ability to maintain them within perceptual recognition. This enables the capacity to understand, integrate, and grasp the significance of perceptual experience and facilitates the processes of symbolization, internal thought, and language development. The dependency upon the evocative qualities of an external object is diminished, and selectivity in the interactions that are sought is strengthened. The mental contents that occupy this sector of transitional space are readily observable by the eye of consciousness.

When the self- and object systems of representation are more effectively united and differentiated by the formation of new mental structures, the skeletal framework for a transitional system of consciousness is outlined. The inner and outer perceptual borders of self-expansion are incorporated in these structures and also develop focused areas of perceptual functioning. It thereby becomes possible to perceive the effects of a given stimulus, from two differing perspectives, simultaneously. Another sector of transitional space is created from the fantasy elaboration of a transitional object that serves well as the mental background for this preconscious system. This psychological space, in being based upon a fantasy, can anchor mental contents that require a greater degree of freedom from the influences of the external world.

The Evolution of Varied Systems of Consciousness

With the dawning of perceptual functioning, a reactive experience is registered when the dormant functions of a primitive ego are awakened. There is insufficient organization within the nuclear self for these body ego experiences, though conscious, to be considered as a system of consciousness. The unconscious realm manifests its activity through the effects of biophysiologic demands upon the nuclear self. The barrier of primal repression reflects the transition from biophysiology to mental representation, and the demands that emanate from this source remain as an unconscious force throughout the life cycle. The transition from an experience of consciousness to an experience reflecting the influence of this unconscious source is determined by the manner in which the continuum of biophysiological demand is registered. An aspect is represented without defense, an aspect is represented with the aid of defense, and an aspect is reacted to as an instinctual impingement with the independent qualities of an object. Although the stimulus is on a continuum of intensity, the early mechanisms of splitting create separate areas of experience. There is as yet no transitional (preconscious) system of consciousness. Ultimately, the buildup of self- and object systems of representations operates as a foundation for the establishment of cohesiveness and continuity of experience. Unifying and differentiating mental structures are formed that incorporate perceptual functions. A gradual process of structural organization, with differing qualities of perception in defined sectors of the personality, delineates a realm of conscious, preconscious, and unconscious mental activities. Increasing quanities of biophysiological demand are capable of representation, and their level of consciousness is reflected by the nature of perception in the varying sectors in which they are registered. Each system of consciousness is regulated by a set of principles that are consonant with their makeup.

A system of consciousness evolves when the boundaries of the self are expanded by the recognition of a separate good object's influence. The resulting transitional space forms a mental background for its contents, which are regulated by the reality principle. In conjunction with the maturation of autonomous ego functions, the development of internal thought, language, and symbolization takes place within this system. It is contained by the perceptual borders of an introjective arm at the pole of the self-representations and a projective arm at the pole of the object representations. The inner border of self-expansion develops a focused area of perceptual activity that functions as the eye of consciousness and determines what is perceived in this sector.

The preconscious system is a realm of mental activity that enables the transition from contents and forces that are unconscious to those that are compatible with consciousness. It is delineated by the structural connections that link the self and object systems of representations, and the fantasy of transitional space (elaborated from the representation of a transitional object) serves as the mental background for its contents. There are two primary structures—the grandiose self and ego ideal—each of which has the capacity to regulate an area of transition. The perceptual borders incorporated in these structures develop focused areas of functioning, which provide the necessary qualities in perception to manage this task.

The grandiose self, based on a fantasy of the object's omnipotence, serves well to regulate mental activity dominated by the pleasure principle. The perceptual border of interior attunement is an integral part of the grandiose self and is capable of perceiving mental contents that are emerging from the unconscious realm. The grandiose self forms the inner border of the preconscious system and develops an area of perceptual activity designed to focus upon the displacements, condensations, and fluid cathectic fluctuations that characterize its mental contents. These contents consist of representations of the self and object, their fantasy elaborations, and nonstructured linkages between them.

The ego ideal, based upon selective identifications, serves well to regulate mental activity dominated by the reality principle. The perceptual border of external attunement is an integral part of the ego ideal and is capable of perceiving the mental contents moving into the conscious realm. The ego ideal forms the outer border of the preconscious system and develops an area of perceptual activity designed to focus upon the logical, linear, sequential ordering of the mental contents entering the conscious system. The grandiose self and ego ideal form the skeletal framework for consolidation of the superego into an independently functioning self-regulatory agency. For this reason, I have referred to this focus of perceptual functioning as the "superego eye."

The boundary for unconscious mental activity must be nonperceptual but reactive in nature. Initially, it was formed by the barrier of primal repression. During the early narcissistic phases of development, it is composed of the structured union of impingements and the reactions to them. Advances in development, leading to a healing of the early splits in the ego, have resulted in the representations of a bad self and bad object being localized at the interior. The impinging aspect of biophysiological demand, represented as a bad instinctual object, mobilizes reactions to impingment, which are represented in the bad self. This connection establishes a rigid, inflexible boundary, which does not allow the evolution of an unconscious system. The effects of unconscious forces exert an influence, but they have not as yet been organized into a system. It is not until genital fantasies of an oedipal conflict have been sufficiently elaborated to exert an organizing influence that the id of the dynamic unconscious can exist as a system of mental functioning.

The pregenital phases of psychosexual development reflect the expanding capacity to represent instinctual demand and the changing conditions of gratification and overstimulation. In a hierarchial fashion, these instinctual body ego experiences and their object-impression counterparts are represented during the height of their predominance. They then recede into the background, as new phases receive emphasis. They will ultimately assume a place in the id of the dynamic unconscous, when a genital consolidation has taken place. There is then a hierarchy of organization, in an unconscious system of mental functioning, ranging from the most primitive oral components to the most advanced oedipal configurations.

The representations of pregenital experience and their fantasy elaborations provide the mental content necessary to utilize instinctual energies having attained varying degrees of neutralization. Their presence facilitates an ongoing process of instinctual integration. Initially, orality predominates making experiences of fusion-merger, envy, greed, and their associated mechanisms of splitting available for use. The shift to anality leaves experiences of sadism, control, and ambivalence in its wake. The ascending hierarchy of organization includes phallic experiences of exhibitionism and voyeurism, before culminating in the unconscious components of gential oedipal experience. The oedipal situation forms new structures at the interior that create a structured pathway of instinctual integration and a new boundary for the unconscious that enables its functioning as a system of mental activity. The resulting id of the dynamic unconscious fosters the process of instinctual integration and provides the means to add depth of meaning to all stimuli.

The Emergence of Repression Proper as the Primary Defense of the Ego

Splitting mechanisms were the principal defensive function that were available in the early phases of development. These translocations of perception enabled the representations of good and bad self-experiences to consolidate and organize into unified entities. When good self-experience was sufficiently structured to heal these early splits, it became possible to register perceptions at their point of impact. Cohesiveness is initiated with the recognition of a separate good object's influence and is stabilized by the formation of the first fixation point on the projective arm of perception. This fixation point is based on the line of continuity of prohibitive experience, which has enabled a recognition of the good object's bad qualities. Cohesiveness is advanced with the formation of the grandiose self and ego ideal, whose structural linkages further unite and differentiate the self- and object systems of representation. A structural foundation is established that will allow repression proper to function as a defensive activity.

The processes of selective identification, involved with the ego ideal, direct perceptual attention into the self-system of representations. A fixation point is formed on the introjective arm of perception that is based on a recognition of the line of continuity of instinctual experience and the good self's bad qualities. There is now sufficient psychic organization for continuity of experience to be viable within the personality. This is a necessary prerequisite because repression proper requires that perceptual attention be directed away from what is most threatening and toward that which is least threatening. The ability to accomplish this complex task is abetted by the organization of a regulatory structure, which is capable of signaling the need for a defensive response and of indicating the area of danger.

In conjunction with the consolidation of the component instincts into a genital drive, the lines of continuity of experience unite to form the structure of castration anxiety. The line of continuity of instinctual experience reflects the gradual shading, from that which is gratifying to that which is overstimulating in self-experience. The line of continuity of prohibitive experience reflects the gradual shading, from that which is restraining to that which is prohibitive and impinging in the influences of an object. This structure, in being made up of the instinctual self-representations (good and bad) and the prohibitive representations of the object (good and bad), is uniquely adapted to serve a signaling and regulating function.

The oedipal situation refers to the elaboration in fantasy of genital instinctual representations. These fantasy linkages particpate in the formation of new structures, which provide the framework for an ever-expanding integration of biophysiologic demands and a new boundary for the unconscious system of mental activity. It is mentioned now to indicate the developmental thrust that is available, when repression proper is well established as a primary defensive response. The stabilizing conditions which have evolved during the pregenital phases, are important for the oedipal conflict to fully flourish and exert its organizing influence. The particular oedipal configuration that is manifested is powerfully affected by gender, as a consequence of the differences in body ego experiences and libidinal objects, especially during the phallic period.

The manner in which the oedipal conflict is shaped, experienced, and resolved will determine the degree of dominance of the reality principle as a governing intrapsychic force. This underscores Freud's (1938/1964) early reflections concerning the reality and pleasure principles. The original ego is a body ego under the influence of reality. It requires a degree of development for the pleasure principle to emerge as a dominant governing principle. Finally, there is a return to the dominance of the reality principle that is initiated with the formation of the ego ideal. The presence of both principles, operating in different sectors of the personality simultaneously, is made possible as a result of the relationship between the grandiose self and the ego ideal.

In the early stages of development, regulation is largely dependent upon interactions with the external world. The object impressions of those interactions are represented to form a functional system that is the foundation for what will become an internal regulator—the superego. The superego is first present as a mental structure, rather than in its component parts or superego nuclei, when the grandiose self and ego ideal form its perceptual boundaries. The mechanism of splitting within the ego that was a part of early development, with the establishment of cohesiveness and continuity of experience, is manifested within the superego. The signaling function of castration anxiety is activated when instinctual demand reaches an intensity beyond the existent regulatory capacities. Repression proper, in its initial stages, utilizes the perceptual functions of the superego eye to direct attention away from the source of a potentially threatening stimulus. The threat may be most evident in the self-system of representations or in the object system of representations, depending upon the particular conditions at the time it is registered. Perceptual attention can then be directed toward the defensive alignments in the alternate system. Repression proper maintains a separation between the representations of good and bad self-experiences and the good and bad influences of an object. The connections that are necessary to insure continuity of experience are embodied in the structure of castration anxiety and expressed in the formation of derivatives. The effective functioning of repression proper is dependent upon the signaling function of castration anxiety and an interrelationship with the evolving superego.

The Structure and Significance of Castration Anxiety

Anxiety is the experience of an internal threat or danger that accompanies each new level of psychic organization. During the pregenital phases of development, it is indicative of a disruptive force and is disorganizing in its effects. Castration anxiety has a specific structure as its foundation that consolidates during the ascendency of phallic and genital instinctual experience. It is unique in that it reflects the presence of a unifying, self-regulatory influence within the personality that is expressed by an anticipation of danger. The underlying structure of castration anxiety is formed by uniting the lines of continuity of experience, instinctual in the self-system of representations and prohibitive in the object system of representations. Thus anxiety is manifested as a consequence of an advancing degree of self-differentiation and individuation that further structuralize and strengthen cohesiveness. Rather than being disruptive, its effects foster integration. Separation–individuation has enabled self-expansion through polarizing two separate systems of representations. Castration anxiety serves to bind the two systems from the surface to the depths and emphasizes the distinction between good and bad qualities. The bonds of continuity of experience are reenforced, making this structure accessible to all aspects of mental representation. It is responsive to any increase in intensity of instinctual demand emanating from the internal world and to the stimuli of expanding interactions with the external world.

The structure of castration anxiety reflects a specific relationship of the self and object, in which the representations of good and bad genital instinctual self-experiences are linked by the fantasy elaborations of a good and bad restraining, prohibitive object's influence. It is then available to operate as a regulator of phallic and genital instinctual activity and to signal the need for defense when the intensity of instinctual demand requires a stronger prohibitive force. The particular composition of castration anxiety and the way it is experienced is unique in each individual, though its regulatory and signaling functions remain the same. There are differences in male and female development that are a product of the differences in the body ego experiences of genital sensations and genital exploration. Prohibitive responses tend to be more defined and castrative in the male and more diffuse and disapproving in the female. This structure is an essential restraining force within the personality, is in a constant state of readiness to institute a defensive response, and its formation is indicative of sufficient self-regulation for the genital oedipal fantasies to flourish.

The Preconditions Necessary for the Elaboration of an Oedipal Conflict

The oedipal conflict is the first expression of an intrapsychic conflict, based upon fantasy, that involves all aspects of self-experience and of an object's influence. This genitally determined conflict can only evolve and flourish when a sequence of phase- and stage-specific developmental tasks have been successfully negotiated. These include the negotiation of a symbiosis, of separation and inividuation, and of the steps preparing for a shift from a narcissistic to an object-related orientation. In the pregenital phases of development, the enhancement and expansion of the self could only take place through the influences of a narcissistic involvement with an object. This is, the object's significance was determined by what it brought to the self. To a greater or lesser degree, there has been a dependency on external objects for the building of psychic structure and for regulatory functions that were deficient. The genital phase of development, initiated with the elaboration of oedipal constellations, is concerned with the formation of new mental structures that enable an object-related orientation. This means that self-expansion can continue by virtue of an object's importance; it is the ability to be involved with an object that enhances the self. Although there continues to be a dependence on external objects to further developmental progression, the nature of the body ego experiences that are needed changes from their earlier narcissistic focus. The more separated, individuated, and differentiated state of the self is associated with internal regulation and an expanded ability to exercise selectivity in the choice of experience. This shift in orientation requires the capacity to perceive an object as having separate and independent objects of its own. The structural consequences of negotiating pregenital developmental tasks provides the preconditions necessary for the genital fantasies of an oedipal conflict to exert this organizing influence.

First, it is important to have structuralized the internal world so that varying systems of consciousness, in continuity with each other, can register the same stimulus with differing levels of meaning. The level of meaning would need to be consonant with the perceptual locale in which the stimulus resonates and the corresponding regulatory principles under which it operates. It is only in this way that the oedipal fantasies can create effects, in the interior of the personality, that are not unduly disruptive to adaptive functions at the periphery. Conversely, perceptual contact with the external world at the periphery of the personality does not unduly interfere with new structure formation at the interior.

An experience of consciousness and a system of consciousness, though they are related phenomena, have a different meaning and significance. The systems of conscious, preconscious, and unconscious mental activities have specific perceptual boundaries and specific principles of regulation. Tracing their evolution and lines of development adds clarity to the manner in which a given stimulus can be perceived and experienced in differing ways simultaneously. The experience of consciousness is present with the onset of perceptual functioning. The form and manner in which the nuclear self registers the effects of stimulation are expressions of consciousness. It is a reactive experience of consciousness, but the defined boundaries or governing principles to define it as a system do not exist. The nuclear self also contains the perceptual barrier of primal repression. This barrier reflects the transition from biophysiology to mental representation and is indicative of demands that are unconscious but insufficiently organized to function as a system.

The delineation of perceptual boundaries, for what will become systems of conscious, preconscious, and unconscious mental activities, is initiated with the process of separation–individuation. The search for, and discovery of, a separate good object's influence form a sector of transitional space for the conscious system and two borders of perceptual attunement to the inner and outer worlds. The grandiose self, a unifying and differentiating structure designed to balance the experience of vulnerability with separateness, incorporates these perceptual borders to form an interior boundary for the preconscious system. The ego ideal, a unifying and differentiating structure designed to strengthen the self-representations through selective identifications, also incorporates these perceptual borders to form an exterior boundary for the preconscious system. The representations of early developmental experience are organizing into a hierarchy that will occupy the id of the dynamic unconscious.

The grandiose self develops focused areas of perceptual activities that enable its function as a boundary and has sufficient instability and involvement with fantasy to allow the pleasure principle and primary process to govern. It has the capacity to regulate the effects of an evolving unconscious system upon preconscious mental activity. The ego ideal also develops focused areas of perceptual activities that enable its function as a boundary and, in being anchored to reality, is uniquely suited to regulate the effects of the reality principle and secondary process. The grandiose self directs perceptual attention inward toward the deeper layers of the preconscious system and outward toward its surface layers. The ego ideal directs perceptual attention inward to the surface layers of the preconscious system and outward to the contents of the conscious system. The eye of consciousness and ego ideal form perceptual boundaries for a conscious system—the ego ideal and grandiose self for a preconscious system. The boundary for an unconscious system must, of necessity, be nonperceptual in nature. During these pregenital phases, it is composed of the representations of impingements and the reactions to them. This boundary does not possess the flexibility necessary for an unconscious system, though it is reactive to unconscious forces. With the emergence of an oedipal constellation, a new boundary will be formed that facilitates the organization of an unconscious system. The formation of these boundaries establishes a continuity of perceptual experience possessing differing qualities that range from contents that are conscious to those that are preconscious and ultimately to those that occupy an unconscious system.

The second precondition necessitates a state of cohesiveness, sufficiently firm, that it can be sustained under the additional stress of linkages that embody conflict. The self- and object systems of representation have been structurally united and differentiated with the formation of the grandiose self and ego ideal. The connection has transpired at the periphery and embodies linkages of good self-experience with the influences of a good object. The representations of bad self-experience and of a bad object's influence are maintained at the interior. Cohesiveness is not fully insured until structural unions can be formed between the two systems in this realm. The oedipal situation is designed to accomplish this developmental task, as the genital fantasies of a bad self and object are structurally united. The stress associated with attaining this new level of psychic organization is intensified by the increase in instinctual activity requiring defense and places the cohesiveness of the self in potential jeopardy. Stage and phase specificities have been essential factors in establishing cohesiveness on a firm enough foundation to support the impact of this new development.

The recognition of separateness evokes an awareness of enormous vulnerability and helplessness. This occurs during the anal period when good instinctual experiences of mastery and control are in the ascendency. A motive is present to create a new structure that can serve the functions of balancing the experience of vulnerability. The stage- and phase-specific mental representations of the self and object provide a perfect match. The optimally gratifying anal object is represented as offering opportunities for mastery and control and is elaborated into fantasies of omnipotence. The representations of good instinctual self-experience are linked by these omnipotent fantasies to the influence of a good instinctual object. The resulting structure is built upon participation in the fantasied omnipotence of an object, and I have referred to it as the "grandiose self."

The aspects of good instinctual self-experience, which are bound into fantasy in forming the grandiose self, are unavailable to respond to the adaptive demands of the external world. In this respect, the self-representational system is depleted, which creates a motive for forming another new structure that can restabilize this system. The stage- and phase-specific mental represntations that are available again provide a perfect match. The representations of autonomous functioning are elaborated into fantasies of those self-potentials that are needed to strengthen the weakened adaptive capacities. The fantasied potentials are linked to the representations of an object's influence that are most needed and hence most admired. The optimally frustrating impressions of a good object are most frequently selected because the depletion in good instinctual self-experience invokes the need for restraint. I have referred to this structure as the "ego ideal" because it is built upon the representation of an object's influence and involves a process of selective identification. The grandiose self and ego ideal, when formed in a stage- and phase-specific manner, unite and differentiate the self- and object systems of representation, to establish cohesiveness on a sound basis. This facilitates an ongoing process of derivative formation that further solidifies cohesiveness and prepares the groundwork for new structures to form at the interior.

The third precondition requires the presence of sufficient stability to contain the increase in instinctual demand associated with a genital expansion and to prevent the disruptive effects of external stimuli from interfering with the formation of new mental structures. Fixation points refer to the effects of perceiving good and bad qualities emanating from a single source of stimulation. The polarization of two separate systems of representations (that are then united and differentiated) has created a projective arm of perception, which is connected to the representations of an object's influence, and an introjective arm of perception extending from the representations of self-experience. The line of continuity of prohibitive experience in the object system and the line of continuity of instinctual experience in the self-system are present as potential perceptual pathways for recognizing these good and bad qualities. When this recognition occurs, a fixation point is established that has a differentiating and regulatory influence based upon the particular infantile attachments that predominate at the time of its formation. The effect is to stabilize cohesiveness, which is necessary when new structures are forming to gain a more advanced degree of psychic organization. However, the memory traces of these infantile attachments continue to exert an influence that must be diminished for new perceptions to be registered with a minimum of distortion.

The initial fixation point, on the projective arm of perception, was based on a recognition of the good object's bad qualities during the anal period. It provided the necessary stability for the grandiose self and ego ideal to form and must remain throughout the life cycle to anchor the representations of an object's influence as a separate system. The anal influence on the continuing object impressions is gradually lessened through processes of depersonification. That is, the original infantile attachment is increasingly symbolized, which serves to strengthen its anchoring function, to facilitate the effectiveness of projective mechanisms, and to enable the inclusion of advancing phallic and genital object impressions.

With the formation of a fixation point on the projective arm of perception, it is still possible for new self-experiences to be registered. The introjective arm of perception remains open for processes of internalization to contribute to the building of psychic structures, which are relatively free of the effects of memory traces. This continues until perceptual attention is directed into the self-system in conjunction with the formation of the ego ideal. The ego ideal is structured with entry into the phallic period of psychosexual development and is associated with a recognition of the good self's bad instinctual qualities. The resulting fixation point on the introjective arm of perception, based upon phallic infantile instinctual experiences, provides the stability necessary for the oedipal situation to structuralize a more advanced level of psychic organization. The stimuli of perceptual contact with the external world are then colored by the memory traces involved in maintaining this point of fixation. A fixed phallic attitude results that, in health, is transient, lasting only until the conflicts engendered by the oedipal situation achieve a resolution. The fixation point on the introjective arm of perception is founded upon the representations of good and bad self-experiences, rather than an infantile attachment to an object. It can thus be readily relinquished when bad instinctual experiences are integrated and no longer require defense. Ultimately, it is essential for the introjective arm of perception to be free of the distorting effects of memory traces, so as to enable the internalization of new experiences from an ever-expanding object-related perspective. This sequence of developmental steps, negotiated in a stage- and phase-specific manner, is preparing the groundwork for a consolidation of the component instincts into a genital drive.

The final precondition that sets the stage for an oedipal constellation to be elaborated in fantasy and exert its organizing influence is the full consolidation of the component instincts into a genitally determined focus. The gradual evolution of the component instincts has reflected an expanding capacity to represent instinctual demand and has focused on those body ego experiences that enable the advancement of increasing degrees of individuation, differentiation, and self-regulation. Each pregenital phase of psychosexual progression has been occupied with an important development step; orality with a symbiosis, anality with separation–individuation, and phallic instinctual interest with preparing for a genital orientation. It is important to maintain a balanced and harmonious interplay of forces during the period of predominance of a given component instinct, so as to not interfere with its stage- and phase-specific functions. The formation of the structure of castration anxiety is a manifestation of a genital consolidation and is indicative of an emerging genital oedipal situation. The representations of the component instincts recede into the interior, where they are organizing to be a part of the id of the dynamic unconscious.

There is now a state of readiness for the seeds of genital experience to rise to the forefront and to be elaborated into the fantasies that comprise the oedipal conflict. The consolidation of the component instincts into a genital drive has created an increase in instinctual activity that is incapable of being represented within a narcissistic organization. Further self-expansion requires a greater capacity to represent the demands of biophysiology, particularly that dimension on the continuum that has been incapable of registration. The genital oedipal fantasies provide linkages that are uniquely suited to unite the self- and object systems, so that a shift from a narcissistic to an object-related orientation can be negotiated. New structures are formed at the interior that ensure the ongoing cohesiveness of the self, establish a continuous pathway for the integration of instinctual demands, and form a new boundary for the unconscious system of mental activity.

An Introduction to the Organizing Influence of the Genital Oedipal Constellation and Its Resolution

The representations of good instinctual self-experience have consolidated to concentrate upon the body ego experiences associated with genital sensations. This perceptual focus upon genital sexuality does not require defense and is elaborated into fantasies of genital involvement as an undamaged (nondefensive) self. The genital instinctual impression of a good object is represented as one that acknowledges genital sexuality, views it as desirable, and recognizes the need for delay until there is sufficient development for the experience to be enhancing with a new and independent object. This imago of optimal gratification includes an optimally frustrating aspect and offers an impression of firm boundaries and restraint. A good object's genitally determined influence is optimally gratifying, in recognizing genital sexuality and presenting an evocative picture of attainment in the future, and is optimally frustrating, in establishing firm limits and regulation. The fantasy elaborations are of mirroring genital effectiveness and restraint. These representations of good qualities of experience are available at the periphery to facilitate adaptive functioning and to bolster the enlarging capacity for instinctual representations. The activity of the autonomous ego functions, represented as a facet of the good self, expands at this locale to form the basis for what will become a conflict-free system. Although there have been areas of functioning that are conflict free, they have not as yet been organized into a system with boundaries and guiding principles. A conflict-free sphere will ultimately form at the periphery, in direct perceptual contact with the external world, when the oedipal conflict is resolved and the superego established as an independent functioning agency.

Genital instinctual experiences that are overstimulating require defense and are represented as a facet of the bad self. These are often associated with masturbatory activities and are elaborated into incestuous fantasies. The dimension on the continuum of instinctual demand that possesses the independent qualities of an object is represented as a genitally overstimulating object. This serves as the portal of entry of instinctual demand and is elaborated into primal scene fantasies.

Incestuous fantasies reflect the defensive responses that are associated with the underlying instinctual experience and are readily linked to the impression of a forbidden instinctual object. When this linkage is structured, the prohibitions that are evoked function as a regulatory force at the interior of the personality. The self- and object systems are thereby united in this locale, establishing cohesiveness on a firmer basis. This defensively constructed, nonperceptual untion forms a reactive barrier that obviates against instinctual activity's gaining direct access to consciousness. It is composed of the more advanced genital impression of an object and linked by a fantasy of bad (defended) genital self-experience. The resulting structure is especially adapted to serve as a new boundary for an unconscious system of mental activity. The previous rigid narcissistic alignment is replaced by this more flexible, object-related boundary, which allows the representations of pregenital experience to be organized into the id of the dynamic unconscious.

Primal scene fantasies reflect the influence of the unseen (un-representable) dimensions on the continuum of biophysiological demand. These genitally determined fantasies are readily linked to self-experiences of overstimulation. When this linkage is structured, an uninterrupted pathway is established that enables instinctual activity to have continuous access to inclusion in the self-system of representations. There is then the potential for exposure to integrative functions, through the line of continuity of instinctual experience. Primal scene fantasies embody the capacity of an unseen instinctual object to evoke body ego experiences of overstimulation. The resulting structure is at the foundation of the ability to attain an object-related perspective. That is, to perceive that an object has independent (unseen) objects of its own. The evolving triadic oedipal configuration is interrelated with the emergence of a structural foundation that secures cohesiveness in a manner that no longer requires a narcissistic orientation. For the first time, it is possible to achieve self-expansion through the significance of involvement with an object.

The organizing influence of the oedipal conflict is set in motion, as the genitally derived lines of continuity of instinctual and prohibitive experience are consolidated into the structure of castration anxiety. The genital fantasies of a bad objects influence and of bad self-experience can then structuralize a foundation that enables continuing self-expansion through object-related experiences. A new level of psychic organization is attained, as the conflicts engendered are resolved through the vehicle of selective identifications. The superego, which has had a line of development at varying levels of organization, can only function as an independent agency when this task has been negotiated.

The perceptual functions of the grandiose self and ego ideal define the outlines of an evolving superego. Their focused areas of perceptual activity create a self-observational function that I have referred to as the "superego eye." Castration anxiety exerts its signaling function by directing perceptual attention away from what is most threatening and toward that which is least threatening. This process of directing perceptual attention away from a source of stimulation is similar to the translocations of perceptions that were necessary during the symbiotic period. The differences are created by the presence of cohesiveness, which establishes continuity of experience in the personality. The early splits in the ego, which fostered the introjection of independent stimuli to build up differentiated self-entities, are healed when the representations of good self-experience are sufficiently consolidated to recognize a separate good object's influence. The splits in the superego, reflecting the functioning of repression proper in the early stages of superego organization, are healed through selective identifications.

The oedipal situation has organized a structured pathway for the integration of instinctual demands. The increase in instinctual activity intensifies the need for selective identifications with those influences of an object that can enhance the self-system of representations. These identifications, along the pathway of the ego ideal, result in a resolution of the oedipal conflict. Instinctual activity reverberates throughout the entire personality and is registered with differing qualities in well-defined systems of consciousness in continuity with each other. The continuing process of selective identification strengthens the self-system, so that the instinctual demand for perceptual attention can be defended against at its source. The splits in the superego are healed, and its regulatory function gains dominance. The superego emerges as an effective independent agency for monitoring the stimuli of the internal and external worlds.

The elaboration and resolution of the oedipal conflict leaves a continuous pathway for the integration of an instinctual demand, from its portal of entry at the interior to attaining secondary autonomy at the periphery. The dimension on the continuum of biophysiological demand that has been potentially most traumatic is registered and represented as a bad instinctual object. A primal scene fantasy is elaborated and is structurally linked to the representation of bad instinctual self-experience. Instinctual demand, though now included within the self-system, possesses overstimulating qualities that evokes the need for a defensive, prohibitive response. However, as the self-system is enhanced by selective identifications, a degree of this instinctual activity no longer requires defense and can be included within the representaitons of good self-experience. Instinctual demand, in having gained access to representation in the good self, has attained secondary autonomy and is available for sublimatory activities.

In conjunction with the resolution of the oedipal conflict, the superego operates in harmony with the interests of the ego, and a conflict-free sphere of functioning is organized at the periphery. The aspects of the self with object qualities that have attained secondary autonomy are available to serve as an inner border, and the representations of empathic experiences, from a new object-related perspective, are becoming available to serve as an outer border. These conditions facilitate the changes in the fixation points that are necessary for further self-expansion to take place.

Fixation points serve as a potential obstacle to new experience. The memory traces at their foundation are evoked by new stimuli and strongly influence or distort the way in which the stimuli are perceived. The fixation points have been essential to provide the stability for the genital oedipal fantasies to flourish during the period of oedipal organization. However, they must undergo changes to enable an influx of new object-related experiences. The fixation point on the introjective arm of perception, based upon the good self's bad qualities, is gradually relinquished in unison with the final step on the pathway of instinctual integration. This arm of perception is the entry point of new stimuli and must be relatively free of the influence of memory traces. The stabilizing function of this fixation point is taken over by the conflict-free sphere. The fixation point on the projective are of perception must remain but be freed of the tenacious influence of the infantile attachments upon which it is based. This is accomplished as these infantile attachments are increasingly symbolized and depersonified. This fixation point is thereby expanded to include the activity of the conflict-free sphere and to broaden the range of mental activities that depend upon projective mechanisms.

Discussion

A's style of communication had shifted. He expressed himself directly to the therapist, with the intent of communicating his inner experiences. This profound change was manifested as A displayed evidence of having developed organized systems of mental representations that were both united and differentiated from each other. A foundation was present that made it possible for him to direct communications to the therapist and not simply react to the interaction.

A's preoccupation with mastery and control was associated with conflict concerning his aggressive drives. The act of self-assertion gave expression to anally derived qualities of good instinctual experience, and he was aware of defensive reactions to the mounting intensity of his poorly regulated anal sadism. Aggression was now capable of being represented as a facet of self-experience. This was in striking contrast to earlier periods of time, when the effects of aggression were disruptive. It only existed in fragmented representations of isolated part self-experience or in isolated impressions of an object. The level of aggression was so overwhelming that it could not be contained, much less be included within the experience of an organized and consolidated self. *A*'s wish to be like General Patton reflected the need for selective identifications that had sufficient restraining force to provide regulation for his aggression. He admired the qualities of a sadistic impinging object and wished to include them within his own adaptive capacities.

A's decision to become aggressive precipitated a body response of severe diarrhea, which was consonant with his lifelong preoccupation with bowel activities. Body ego experiences associated with bowel functions had been utilized to represent instinctual activity (the Make-A-Dos). *A* gradually gained some integration of, and perspective upon, his aggressive drives. This was expressed by laughter at the idea of his rage spilling out in diarrhea. Aggression gradually became less threatening, as *A* developed an increasing capacity to form derivatives. This also made it possible for him to define the nuances and characteristics of his conflict, and he became more effective in establishing mastery and control. Superego nuclei of a prohibitive object's influence were consolidated and could function as a restraining force. This resulted in a feeling of shame and embarrassment at his explosive outbursts.

Aggression was more contained and regulated, and instinctual expansion progressed into the phallic realm. *A*'s phallic exhibitionism emerged and with it, a preoccupation with genital sensations. Concern over the integrity of his penis gave some indication that the structure of castration anxiety was organizing and was capable of a signaling function. This was in contrast to A's earlier experiences with anxiety. When A's autistic position was relinquished, he was overcome by an anxiety of panic proportions; with separation it threatened fragmentation and, associated with his aggressive drives, it was often crippling and debilitating. Anxiety was now appearing as a regulatory force within his personality.

A displayed an ability to be assertive with the therapist, directly expressed his awareness of the therapist's lapse in empathy, and experienced himself as being effective in the interaction. He correctly sensed the therapist's discomfort with his phallic exhibitionism. A's concern over the intactness of his penis was evoked by the therapist's defensiveness. The therapist's validation of A's perception was followed by the recall of a dream, which was the first dream he had reported. The act of communicating a dream was a further manifestation of the more differentiated state of his representational world and of an increased ability to form derivative expressions of meaning. The very structure of a dream embodies the representations of a self, an object, and a linkage between them.

This dream portrayed the effects of the therapeutic interaction and of the integration that had transpired. The image of the old building, which was torn down in order to construct a new building, gave emphasis to the new structures that had formed within A. The old rundown shack was reminiscent of his shattered and fragmented psychic organization and reflected the devastating effects of his experiences during the earliest periods of development. The construction of the new building had reached the thirteenth floor, and A was now in his thirteenth year. The image of a tall new building also seemed to represent the sense of intactness of his erect penis and of sufficient stability to allow instinctual expansion to include phallic and genital dimensions. The search for the top of the building was the first indication that A was thinking of a time when the therapeutic work would come to a conclusion. The dream indicated that this was not yet in sight; the top was not visible. The fact that A could engage in the search indicated an increasing ability to conceive of himself as being separate and individuated.

A's psychic functioning revealed the differing levels of perception that were now available to him. In order to perceive and communicate the contents of his inner world, he had to maintain a simultaneous perception of the immediacy of his responses to the therapeutic interaction and of the derivatives it evoked. This task requires a psychic organization with two separate but continuous levels of perceptual activity. *A* could perceive the contents of his conscious system, and at the same time there was an inner level of focused perceptual activity that identified derivative associations. This appeared to support the idea that focused areas of perceptual activity occur at two separate locales within the personality. The concept of an eye of consciousness focusing perception upon the contents of the conscious system, as well as a superego eye focusing perception upon the contents of the preconscious system, was useful in understanding this new development in *A*. It was possible to observe the gradual organization of differing realms of mental activity. The effects of unconscious mental activity evoked derivatives in the preconscious system, which were on a continuum with the immediate perceptions that occupied the conscious system. The emergence of these varying qualities of perception in *A*, was accompanied by communicative expressions reflecting differentiated unions between the representations of self-experience and the impressions of an object. His expanded capacity to represent instinctual demands was associated with a more organized system of restraint. There was no evidence, to this point, of an oedipal configuration. However, the preconditions that establish a foundation for genital fantasies to exert an organizing influence were forming.

   H and *G* both indicated, in their perceptions of the therapeutic interaction, the effects of maintaining a fixation point on the introjective arm of perception. All stimuli were affected by the infantile experiences that were at the foundation of this fixed manner of perception. *H* stated that it made no difference what the therapist said or did; she would experience the interaction in exactly the same way. It was only when the therapist could respond to the unconscious communication, expressed in her fixed character attitude, that it was possible for *H* to relinquish that defensive fixated perception. She then communicated the derivatives that expressed her manner of representing instinctual activity. These instinctual derivatives revealed the intense conflict that was associated with phallic instinctual activity. The therapist's interpretation that *H* seemed to want help in exploring her body and its inner parts was followed by a diminution in the defensive interference with instinctual experience. *H* revealed that her phallic exhibitionism did not require defense and was represented as an aspect of good self-experience. However, it quickly escalated to an intensity that was overstimulating. Anxiety arose and functioned to signal for a defensive response, which was indicative of a genital consolidation. The resulting structure of castration anxiety mobilized feelings of inadequacy and defectiveness in response to instinctual arousal. This illustrated the difference in the composition of this structure in male and female development. Castration anxiety is based upon the genital representations of an instinctually aroused self, threatened by a prohibitive object. In *H*, the threat was of exposing her inadequacies, whereas in *A* it was of damage to his genitals. The differences were created by differences in the body ego experiences of genital exploration. In *G* the experience of genital overstimulation was accompanied by an intense fear of castration. His association to the circumcision of his infant brother gave expression to this underlying regulatory and signaling structure.

H and *G* exhibited pathological disturbances that resulted from conflict engendered by the genital fantasies of an oedipal constellation. *H* described an instinctual attachment to her mother with genital qualities indicative of a negative oedipal configuration. There were also reverberations to earlier oral attachments that exerted a regressive pull, which underlined the significance of an orderly stage- and phase-specific progression of instinctual representation for a healthy outcome. She also displayed some movement toward displacing her genital interest to a male figure, which was associated with conflict and anxiety. *G* described a genital instinctual attitude toward his mother so fraught with overstimulation and the threat of castration that it could only be managed by developing a symptom of impotence. He recreated the genital conflicts, associated with instinctual arousal, in the transference.

H and *G* also displayed areas of healthy functioning. *H*, in expressing her phallic exhibitionism and genital arousal through masturbatory actions, was able to diminish the inhibitory effects of defensive responses. She could then suspend the dominant (and defensive) perceptual activity of the eye of consciousness and allow the focused perceptual activity of the superego eye to dominate. Derivatives of unconscious instinctual demands then became more accessible. These were expressed in her associations to the guard at the tollbooth who frightened her, in her memories of sexual play, and in the excitement of exploring caves and jungles. *G* was gradually able to relinquish his fixed characterological attitude, as the representations of bad self-phallic and genital experiences upon which they were based became integrated. These instinctual experiences were revived in the therapeutic relationship, were exposed to more advanced areas of psychic functioning, and no longer required defense. The consequence was in a dissolution of his symptom of impotence. *H* and *G* had both negotiated pregenital developmental tasks, but the conflicts of the oedipal situation had interfered with further progression. *H*, at 8 years of age, was displaying the effects of an inability to resolve an overwhelming oedipal conflict. *G* had established a lifelong characterological fixation, necessitated by an unresolved oedipal conflict. In both, the fixation point on the introjective arm of perception, which is transiently fixated during healthy development, was defensively maintained.

The evolution of differing qualities of perception, in differing sectors of the personality, was possible to observe during the course of *A*'s treatment. These qualities of perception had already been established in *H* and *G*. With *A*, it was also possible to trace the manner in which instinctual activity was increasingly represented, as the phases of psychosexual development were unfolding. This could only be inferred with *H* and *G*. It did appear that aggression, in *H* and *G*, was well regulated and differentiating in its effects and that instinctual representation was dominated by phallic and genital experiences. In addition, there was evidence that oral libidinal overstimulation had interfered with a smooth progression to a genital consolidation and contributed to the difficulty.

CHAPTER 7

The Oedipal Conflict as a Psychic Organizer

Introduction

Throughout the history of psychoanalysis, the oedipal conflict has occupied a central position in a metapsychology devoted to the understanding of psychic processes and mental events. The oedipal conflict has also been a focus of disagreements and of causing differing psychoanalytic schools of thought to split off from the main body of classical psychoanalytic metapsychology. Although other factors may have been involved, the disagreements were based upon clinical observations and the manner in which they were understood. For example, Kleinian psychology portrayed the oedipal conflict as being manifested in the earliest stages of an individual's life history. This concept raised much controversy. The basic argument revolved around whether a young infant could have the mental capacity to effect the complex symbolic and representational tasks that are embodied in an oedipal conflict. There is no question that, in primitively organized patients of all ages, there are highly defended mental impressions of an object's possessing instinctual qualities. This same mental impression of an instinctual object is also present in the very early stages of development. However, the meaning attributed to this observation is another matter, as is the task of reconciling this observation with the complex processes involved in an oedipal conflict. In addition, there are some patients whose early development has been profoundly disturbed, in which there is little or no indication of an oedipal conflict.

Clinical evidence seems to indicate that the mental impressions of an instinctually overstimulating object are registered very early in life. These object impressions are represented as posing a threat to any libidinal attachment to a good object's influence. In my opinion, these triangular configurations have been a source of confusion when they are presented as evidence of an oedipal conflict. They can be described as the mental precursors of what will eventually become an oedipal conflict, which places them in a different perspective.

In this presentation, the oedipal conflict refers specifically to the fantasy elaborations of genital representations of self-experience and of an object's influence and of the structural unions that are formed between them. The emergence of this genitally determined intrapsychic conflict is associated with a profound shift, from a narcissistic to an object-related orientation. An object-related experience requires a capacity to perceive the object as having independent objects of its own and is essential for the full flowering of an oedipal conflict. A complex psychic organization is necessary in order to establish that perception of an object, and it is difficult to conceive of an oedipal conflict at any point prior to its existence. To do so is to confuse the precursors with the conflict itself. My impression has been that the oedipal conflict serves a vital organizing function, which is essential for developmental progression to continue beyond the state of narcissism.

In working with a variety of patients over a number of years, two observations consistently emerged that were puzzling to me. One involved the universal presence of the mental impressions of a primal scene experience. In some individuals, the impact of the primal scene was extremely traumatic and played a significant role in influencing the pathology that was present or was a significant aspect of the pathology itself. There were others, for whom what I called a primal scene was not only not traumatic but was frequently associated with an alleviation of anxiety. In addition, there were patients who never offered any validation of having had direct or indirect perceptual contact with the sexual activity of significant others. Yet these same patients displayed instinctual derivatives reflective of a primal scene experience. This could easily be explained as a function of repression, and it may have been. The universality of the phenomena made me wonder if there were some internal event with primal scene significance that was then evoked by the actual experience with external objects.

The second observation that seemed curious to me was the expression of open incestuous fantasies in the absence of anxiety. This also could be explained in a variety of ways. It could be a consequence of the mechanism of isoltation or of the emergence into a consciousness of what had previously been repressed.

I began to reconsider what I had thought of as primal scene material and slowly realized that there was an area of confusion. The experiences that were associated with anxiety all involved an unseen sexual situation. There was a feeling of sexual arousal that was both exciting and frightening, but the objects whose presence was sensed were unseen. These primal scene experiences, though accompanied by anxiety, were expressed within the transference relationship in a manner that facilitated integration. Those situations, which involved a sexual scene with the objects clearly visible, were associated with a heightening of the effects of repression and were expressed in the transference relationship in a manner that obviated against their integration. I had labeled these as ''primal scene derivatives,'' but they could be more fully understood as having incestuous meaning. It became apparent that there was an important distinction to be made between primal scene and incestuous fantasies, in order to determine the significance of both.

When I made this distinction, it appeared evident that derivatives embodying a visualized sexual scene, with incestuous objects, were accompanied by an ascendency of repressive forces. Openly incestuous fantasies were expressed in conjunction with a chain of associations reflective of defensive interference with instinctual experience. Those derivatives that embodied a sexual situation with the objects unseen were associated with instinctual arousal, were accompanied by anxiety, and were expressed in conjunction with a chain of associations reflective of a freer flow of instinctual experience. The effects of repression were less in evidence.

The differences between incestuous and primal scene derivatives seemed to be based upon underlying structures that had evolved from the oedipal conflict. Incestuous fantasies reflected a union between the self and object that had established a firm boundary for unconscious mental activity. Primal scene fantasies reflected a union between the self and object that had established a pathway by which instinctual demand was more fully included within the realm of self-experience. These new structures offered greater stability, insured cohesiveness, and were an integral part of the capacity for object relatedness.

In this chapter, I will discuss the significance of the shift from narcissism to object relatedness and the role of the oedipal conflict as a psychic organizer.

Clinical Material

A's preoccupation with phallic and genital experiences continued. Masturbatory activities surfaced periodically during the course of a given session but gradually abated as his concerns were increasingly verbalized. A had seen his mother undressing and was startled at seeing her without a penis. Many sessions were occupied with anxious questions and repetitive expressions of fantasies, fears, and curiosity. He was startled at the realization that women and girls had no penis. He thought everyone had one and could not imagine someone without one. He was unable to see it, which meant that it had to be in a hidden place. This instigated a flurry of fantasies about, and an intense preoccupation with, the reproductive process that was interspersed with fragments of information he had learned in school. It was hard for him to grasp the information he had been given. He thought babies grew inside of a penis and were born in that fashion. He had learned about the relationship of sexual intercourse and reproduction in school and repeatedly attempted to reconcile what he had learned with his extreme difficulty in thinking of a penis entering the inside of a woman. He would then giggle as he imagined a penis entering a man, either anally or orally. His attitude, when he thought of this genital union, was one of excitement intermingled with anxiety. His attitude, in imagining a penis entering a woman, was one of very intense anxiety. It was expressed in a frantic, rigid, stereotyped repetition of the idea. He was attempting to master the idea with his thinking process.

The following session occurred after an hour in which A had talked of his increasing awareness of girls in his environment. He had spoken of how mysterious and exciting they seemed to him and expressed his fearful concern as to how he could possibly initiate a sexual contact. The session began with the therapist's being 2 minutes late. *A* had noticed the time and was extremely upset at having to wait. While anxiously waiting, he had fantasied that the therapist was talking with his wife. He felt his anxiety mount as he looked at the closed door and became increasingly upset as his time came and the door remained closed. The therapist stated his lateness had threatened to rupture the bond between them, and it felt to *A* that a woman had pulled the therapist away from him. *A* responded by talking of the various girls he had come in contact with. He did not know how to talk to them and felt paralyzed. He was becoming increasingly interested but felt immobilized in knowing what to say or how to approach them. He desperately wanted to reach out and felt totally lost in knowing how. The therapist stated that he was reminded of Pa-Ba, the helpless infant. Pa-Ba had needed a mother desperately, and the mothering he found had crippled him. *A* became silent and appeared preoccupied. He remained in silent contemplation for an extended period of time. His face suddenly lit up, and he described a trip that he had taken to explore a cave. Some of the rooms were extremely large, some were small and narrow. The largest room was lit so that the dimensions of the cave could be seen. A guide turned off the lights to show what total darkness was like. When the lights were off, *A* felt a sense of danger. The guide then turned on a flashlight and pointed out the various openings that led deeper into the earth. *A* felt safe exploring the cave with the guide but was frightened when he thought of exploring it alone.

I, a very thin 22-year-old unmarried woman, was in great distress. Her symptom of vomiting prevented her from many desired activities. She could never go out to eat because she feared she might vomit and be extremely humiliated. On those occasions when she went out, she was preoccupied with her fear of being humiliated. She also felt that she was not living up to her capacities. She worked as a secretary, had avoided further education, and regretted it. At work she felt unhappy and was plagued by a silent attachment to an older man. She felt intensely jealous in hearing any talk of his family. She was terrified of heterosexual relationships. She was frequently sought out by men her age and always avoided this contact.

The patient spent the first months of her treatment talking relatively freely of her life, her experiences in growing up, and of her wishes and aspirations. Verbalizations by the therapist were experienced by her as infantalizing or as an interference. A comment or question by the therapist would instigate a dream in which some obstacle interfered with her progress. She appeared most comfortable in the therapist's silence. Her father had been in the armed services during the first 3 years of her life. Two siblings were born, 1 and 3 years after his return. She spoke of her mother with much contempt, stressing her subjugation to her husband and lack of aspirations for herself. She implicitly, and derivatively, communicated an intense feeling of closeness to her mother and was uneasy as to its erotic significance. She strictly adhered to a perception of the therapist as a listening and helping figure.

I began to have a series of openly incestuous dreams, in which she was involved in a sexual relationship with her father. Her attitude in reporting the dreams was one of mild curiosity and puzzlement as to how she could have such inner experiences. The following session occurred immediately afterwards. *I* entered, lay on the couch, and began to feel an intense itching on her inner thigh. She spoke of it with great embarrassment and hesitation. She wanted to scratch but felt immobilized in the therapist's presence. The sensation built in intensity until she had to scratch it. As she did, she recalled how little she knew of sexual matters. She remembered the shock of her first menstrual period. It was not the blood but the realization of an opening in her body that she had no idea existed. She became restless and for the first time expressed a desire for the therapist to talk. Previously, the therapist's words were unwanted, and there had not even been the most minimal question or request. The wish to hear the therapist's words mounted, "Why won't you talk?" She went on to hesitantly express her fear that the therapist thought she was masturbating. She knew this had never been a part of her life. She has heard others speak of it, but in no way had she engaged in such a practice. She recalled being teased as a child for going to the bathroom so frequently and then described her driven efforts to wipe herself. She noticed a similarity to the itching sensation. The request for the therapist's words escalated to a demand, "Won't you talk!" The therapist stated that, as she itched, she also felt an intense longing for him to bring something to her to relieve her itch. It looked as though those two sensations were connected. She began to giggle and to cry. She just thought of a silly joke she heard when she was small. She wanted to laugh, even though what it meant did not seem funny. "I feel like I'm the hot dog bun and you are the hot dog." The patient became silent and noticed that the feeling in her throat, initiating an episode of vomiting, was an itching sensation. When she scratched the inside of her thigh, she thought of her throat and became aware of sensations in her genitals. *I* then recalled the previous day. She had left her gloves in the therapist's office and had returned to get them. The door was closed, and she knew the therapist was with someone. She felt both excited and terrified. Her anxiety increased; she quickly turned and left and tried to put it out of her mind.

The Shift from Narcissism to Object Relatedness

During the pregenital phases of development, a narcissistically determined perceptual focus has been essential in order to build up functional systems of representation that can be united and differentiated. The primary thrust for developmental progression is motivated by the need for an expanding capacity to represent the demands of biophysiology, within a psychic organization that is insufficiently structured and stabilized to regulate the impact. The evolution of the component instincts is reflective of the phases of narcissistic experiences that are necessary to accomplish this task.

The body ego experiences that predominate during a given period are consonant with the level of psychic organization that is available and the developmental step that must be negotiated. Stage and phase specificity is essential, in order to enable expanding areas of instinctual experience to make their unique contribution toward advances in psychic structuralization. Initially, the experience is orally determined, which fosters the introjective processes necessary to consolidate self-entities and prepare for separation and individuation. During the anal phase, narcissistic interest centers upon the experiences of mastery and control that are essential for a successful outcome of the process of separation–

individuation. The phallic phase serves to consolidate narcissistic interest, stabilize the recently acquired state of cohesiveness, and highlight the genital as the symbolic organ of connection to an object. The capacity for strengthening the self-system of representations, through including the admired influences of an object, has been established. The component instincts are consolidated into a genital drive, which sets the stage for the formation of an oedipal conflict.

A narcissistic perspective has been essential for the expansion of the component instincts, and for developing a mental foundation that can utilize the perception of an independent object's influence to further self-expansion. In a narcissistically structured personality, the increase in instinctual activity associated with a genital orientation is threatening and potentially traumatic. With the attainment of a genital consolidation, this narcissistic organization is placed in a phobic situation. A motive is present that stimulates the formation of new structures, which are designed to enhance the capacity for instinctual representation. These new structures develop from the linkages provided by the genital instinctual fantasies that comprise an oedipal conflict.

Developmental progression has reached a point where a shift is required, from a narcissistic to an object-related orientation. For the first time, it is possible for an object-related perceptual experience to be potentially enhancing. The continuum of biophysiological demand has a dimension possessing the independent qualities of an object and a dimension that has been unrepresentable. The oedipal situation creates the psychological wherewhithal to perceive that which has previously been unseen and to include within the realm of self-experience that which has previously been reactively excluded. The sequence of developmental steps negotiated during the pregenital, narcissistic phases has made it possible to gain a new perception of the stimuli of the internal and external worlds. An oedipal situation requires the ability to perceive an object as having independent (unseen) objects of its own and operates to structuralize that perception. A phobic situation has set in motion the elaboration of genitally determined fantasies that will ultimately result in a new object-related psychic organization.

The oedipal situation necessitates a genital orientation and utilizes the representations of all aspects of self-experience and of an object's influence to exert its organizing function. It includes an intrapsychic conflict that could be given any name. The myth of Oedipus captures the composition of the genital fantasy elaborations, in the realm of bad experience at the interior, that participate in the formation of new structures insuring object-related perceptions. An object-related perception includes a genital sexual awareness of the primary love object and with it the associated experience of sexual rivalries and jealousies. Body ego experiences of excitement and danger emerge from this new way of perceiving stimuli and interactions. Potentialities are opened up, and with them an expanded capacity to perceive the nuances and complexities of relationships. The external object, previously perceived only in regard to its narcissistic significance, can now be seen with an awareness of triadic and multiadic relationships. A careful study of the emerging oedipal constellation, its function as a psychic organizer, and its resolution can aid in discriminating its healthy and pathological manifestations.

The Relationship of Castration Anxiety to the Emerging Oedipal Constellation

With the consolidation of the component instincts, the seeds of genital experience are intensified and expand. The lines of continuity of instinctual and prohibitive experience are united to form the structure of castration anxiety. Cohesiveness, which has been structuralized at the periphery by the grandiose self and ego ideal, is strengthened by this linkage that reaches from the periphery and extends toward the interior. This structure serves a regulatory function and is uniquely adapted to signal for the institution of a defensive response with the slightest unmanageable increase in instinctual demand. It is composed of the representations of good and bad instinctual self-experiences and the good and bad restraining, prohibitive impressions of an object; it operates within the realm of preconscious mental activity and is responsive to the effects of unconscious mental activity. It is possible to maintain a

constant state of readiness to institute defense because representations of the self and object, both good and bad, and of instinctual activity and prohibition are included. Castration anxiety
regulates the influx of intinctual demand from the interior and the
effects of stimuli from the external world.

Genital instinctual experiences that do not require defense are
more freely available, when linked to the optimally frustrating impressions of a good object that provides an inner presence of restraint. Optimally frustrating impressions of a good object are on
a line of continuity of prohibitive experience and shade into the
impinging impressions of a bad object. Thus, when genital instinctual activity is heightened and reaches levels of intensity that are
overstimulating, the castrative prohibitive threats of a bad object's
influence are invoked.

In the initial stages of genital instinctual expansion, perceptual
attention is directed toward defensively organized responses and
away from the source of a stimulus. However, because cohesiveness is established and continuity of experience ensured, a connection to the source is maintained through the formation of
instinctual derivatives. The derivatives are composed of appropriate representations of self-experience, of an object's influence, and
of the linking fantasy that expresses resonance with the source of
a stimulus. The increasing complexity of interactions with varied
objects in the external world evokes the activity of instinctual
derivatives and provides depth and meaning to an enlarging range
of relationships. The formation of instinctual derivatives is intimately interrelated with the signaling and regulatory functions of
castration anxiety, which further solidifies continuity of experience
within the personality.

The Oedipal Situation

The Relationship to the Systems of Consciousness

The consolidation of instinctual activity into a genital focus
reflects the expanding capacity to represent instinctual demand
and exerts an effect upon conscious, preconscious, and unconscious experiences. During the narcissistic phases of development,

the mental impression of a bad instinctual object was reacted to as an impingement. Prior to the shift from narcissism to object relatedness, the boundary for an unconscious system was formed by this union. The line of continuity of instinctual experience was thereby interrupted, due to the degree of defensive activity that was necessary. That line of continuity consists of the representations of good instinctual self-experience shading into bad instinctual self-experience as defenses are required and extending to the impression of a bad instinctual object (the portal of entry of instinctual demand). The recognition of the good self's bad qualities establishes a fixation point on the introjective arm of perception, which creates the stability required for the structure of castration anxiety to consolidate and for the genital fantasies comprising the oedipal situation to flourish. The oedipal conflict refers to the specific genital fantasies, elaborated in the realm of bad experience at the interior, that instigate an intrapsychic conflict of opposing forces. These fantasies function to form new structures that enable the capacity for object-related perceptions.

The impression of a bad instinctual object is elaborated into a genital primal scene fantasy that is structurally linked to the representations of bad genital, instinctual self-experience. The portal of entry of instinctual demand is no longer present as the stimulus for maintaining mental contents within the unconscious realm of activity. A structured pathway of integration is formed that makes the total continuum of biophysiological demands, including its unseen dimensions, accessible to representation within the self-system. This is the intrapsychic equivalent of perceiving the independent qualities of an external object. The shift to an object-related perceptual orientation requires the formation of a new boundary for the unconscious system. It must be a nonperceptual structure capable of excluding disruptive mental content and be reactively associated with derivatives that are resonant with an expression of their meaning. When the representations of bad instinctual self-experience are elaborated into genital incestuous fantasies and linked to the representation of a bad instinctual object, the resulting structure forms a new object-related boundary for the unconscious system. It is a more flexible boundary, is associated with derivatives expressive of unconscious mental content, and provides defensive regulation for the continuing influx of instinctual demand. The structuralization of these genitally determined oedipal linkages unites the self- and object systems of representation at the interior and solidifies cohesiveness. The result is in a regulated increase in the dimensions of biophysiological demand that can be represented and an expanded perceptual capacity that includes the recognition of an object's having independent objects of its own.

The grandiose self and ego ideal form boundaries for the transition from unconscious to conscious mental activity that defines the preconscious system. The focused area of perceptual functions that are incorporated in the structure of the grandiose self registers the effects of the unconscious system upon preconscious mental activity. This structure is involved with fantasy and is unstable enough to regulate the influence of primary process activity upon the preconscious system. The focused area of perceptual functions incorporated in the structure of the ego ideal registers the effects of preconscious mental activity upon the conscious system. The ego ideal is involved with external reality and is stable enough to regulate the influence of secondary process activity.

The ascendancy of the genital experiences comprising an oedipal situation, as well as the associated development of object-related perceptions, is the final step in the organization of an id of the dynamic unconscious. For the first time, the unconscious system is composed of a hierarchy of mental representations that range from those of the most primitive stages to those that have defined a new nonperceptual boundary. Thus, in the most advanced stage of organization, genital experiences will be at the boundary of preconscious mental activity. The primitive representations of early experiences of orality will be more deeply embedded in the unconscious system, closer to the realm of biophysiology and the border of primal repression. The id of the dynamic unconscious is a structured system of mental activity, composed of the representations of an advancing hierarchy of narcissistic developmental experiences. These provide the wherewithal for utilizing instinctual energies, with varying degrees of neutralization, to evoke the formation of derivations. This is the vehicle by which unconscious mental activity exerts its effect upon preconscious and conscious experiences.

The source of stimulation may arise at the interior from the continuum of biophysiologic demand (the self with object qualities) or result from perceptual contact with the external world (the object with self-qualitiies). The nature of the experience varies as the stimulus resonates throughout the personality and is perceived at differing levels of psychic organizations that are in continuity with each other. The realm of mental activity in which a stimulus is registered, the mental structures that occupy that realm and the principles that govern their functions, and the nature of the focused perceptual activity determine the meaning of the experience.

The consolidation of the component instincts into a genital drive has highlighted the awareness of genital sensations. Those that do not require defense are represented as a facet of good self-experience, which, along with the influences of a good instinctual object, occupy the conscious system. The fixation point on the introjective arm of perception is based on a recognition of the gradual shading of good instinctual self-experience into bad instinctual self-experience, as defenses are instituted. This also reflects the transition from the conscious to the preconscious system. The representations of bad self-experience and of a bad object's influence are at the boundary of the unconscious system, and it is their fantasy elaborations that constitute an oedipal conflict. The new structures that are formed maintain the boundary and create a continuous pathway for the influx and integration of instinctual demand. The pathway is not complete until a resolution of the conflict is attained. At that point, instinctual demand can move without undue interference from its portal of entry in the unconscious system, to inclusion within the representations of bad self-experience in the preconscious system, to being exposed to integrative forces so as to no longer require defense and gain entry into the conscious system. The latter step is equivalent to attaining secondary autonomy and is associated with the dissolution of the fixation point on the introjective arm of perception; that is, as instinctual activity that was represented as a part of the bad self is included within the good self, the punitive effects of castration anxiety are modified and the fixation point is relinquished.

The representations of a good object's influence, which is located within the conscious system, have been utilized to form the grandiose self and ego ideal. These differentiating structures are extended to form boundaries for the transitions from unconscious to preconscious, and preconscious to conscious, mental activities.

They regulate the formation of derivatves in the preconscious and unconscious systems and are organizing into the independent agency of the superego. The line of continuity of prohibitive experience reaches into all levels of consciousness, from the representations of optimal frustration in the conscious system, shading into prohibitions in the preconscious system, to instinctually influenced impingements within the unconscious system. The ego ideal, formed by selective identifications, has established a perceptual pathway that enables the influences of an object to be included within the self-system of representations. The increase in instinctual activity accompanying the oedipal situation creates a greater need, in the self-system, for the exercise of restraint and prohibition. A powerful motive is present to strengthen the self-system, through accelerating the process of selective identification. This is the vehicle for achieving a resolution of the oedipal conflict, which eventuates in the superego's consolidating as an independently functioning intrapsychic agency. When the need for restraint is excessive, it is the prohibitive and impinging influences of objects that are admired. This process of identification with an aggressor is the mechanism by which the prohibitive functions of the superego are manifested within the self-system of representations.

The oedipal constellation serves to insure cohesiveness and continuity of experience within the personality, by strengthening the various connections between all aspects of the functional systems of representation. Repression proper can then ascend as the primary defensive activity of the ego that, in monitoring and censoring mental content, enables well-defined systems of consciousness to be present in continuity with each other.

The Effect upon the Self- and Object Representational Systems

Genital instinctual expansion has an organizing influence upon the functional systems of representation. The discrete entities of good and bad selves and objects are bound together more effectively, so as to enhance stability and anchor object constancy. Selective identifications involve the good self and good object, identifications with an aggressor, the bad object and good self, the line of continuity of instinctual experience, the good and bad selves, and the new structures forming at the interior, the bad self and bad object. Each of these connections is interrelated with the others; this facilitates their specific functions.

During the pregenital, narcissistic phases of development, lines of continuity of experience have been present within the personality, in a form that is readily disrupted. These lines of continuity maintain a connection between the representations of good and bad qualities of experience that must be strengthened for object constancy and object relatedness to be viable and secure.

The representations of good self-experience include the activity of the autonomous ego functions, the background object of primary identification, and phase-specific instinctual gratifications. The representations of bad self-experience include sensory deprivations, reactions to impingement, and intinctual overstimulation. The good and bad self-entities are thus connected by this line of continuity of instinctual experience, as an increasing intensity shades into overstimulation. No other facet of self-experience has this quality. It is a manifestation of the effects on perception of the self with object qualities. The dimension not requiring defense is registered within good self-experience, and the dimension requiring defense within bad self-experience. This connection is stabilized by the formation of a fixation point in preparation for an oedipal conflict and is strengthened as instinctual experience is integrated with its resolution. The dimension on the continuum of biophysiological demand, incapable of representation within the self-system, is registered with the impression of a bad instinctual object. It is this extension of the line of continuity of instinctual experience that is structuralized, during the oedipal period, to enable an uninterrupted flow of instinctual demand from the interior to the periphery. A firm bond is established between the bad self and bad object that ensures cohesiveness at the interior.

The representations of a good object's influence include impressions of a transitional object, of optimal gratification, and of optimal frustration. The representations of a bad object's influence include impressions of sensory deprivation, of instinctual overstimulation, and of impingements. The good and bad object entities are connected by a line of continuity of prohibitive experience, as the restraint associated with optimal frustration shades through prohibitions into impingements. Thus instinctual experience resonates throughout the personality from the interior to the periphery, whereas restraining forces resonate from the periphery to the interior. The structure of castration anxiety, which consolidates the lines of continuity of instinctual and prohibitive experience, serves to more firmly anchor object constancy and unify the separate self- and object entities. The signaling and regulatory functions of castration anxiety are essential for the genital fantasies of the oedipal conflict to flourish. They provide prohibitive influences that range from the gentle restraint evoked by good genital instinctual experiences, to the impinging threat of castration evoked by genitally overstimulating experiences. In maintaining a connection of the good and bad selves to the good and bad objects, they are in a state of readiness for any stimulus to be capable of activating a defensive response.

The id of the dynamic unconscious is established as a system of mental activity, when the genitally determined incestuous fantasies are structured to form its boundary. It is composed of the representations of narcissistic experience, organized in a hierarchy, that reflects the advancement of the component instincts. They are available at varying levels of organization to enable the primary process to hold sway and consist of those qualities of bad experience too disruptive to gain access to consciousness and those qualities of good experience too primitive to occupy other sectors of the personality. Instinctual movement through the id of the dynamic unconscious is a passage through the narcissistic developmental history of the individual and initiates the process of integration. The representations of bad self-experience always involve body ego experiences of overstimulation. The nature of the overstimulation is shaped by the particular psychosexual phase in which it occurs. During the oral phase, it is of greed, elaborated into cannibalistic fantasies. The anal experience is of loosely bound libidinal and aggressive drives, elaborated into sadistic fantasies. The phallic experience is of overstimulation in looking and being looked at, elaborated into voyeuristic fantasies. In the genital phase, the body ego experience of masturbatory overstimulation is elaborated into incestuous fantasies. These fantasies serve a linking function by including an object. A structural linkage is effected with the representation of a bad instinctual object, establishing the genital instinctual representation of the bad self as the most advanced in the hierarchy of the id of the dynamic unconscious. A genital instinctual orientation requires repression proper to be operative and monitored by the structure of castration anxiety. The process of genital instinctual integration is facilitated by its powerful regulatory and signaling functions. The representations of bad self-experiences can only form unions with the impressions of a bad object under these conditions. The whole bad self is thus located at the boundary of the unconscious system, and the other facets of bad self-experiences are accessible in the preconscious system to participate in defensive responses.

The body ego experience of sensory deprivation is an experience of unrealized potentials. The autonomous ego functions are amplified by empathic resonance from contact with an external object and through their use in adaptive tasks. The representations of sensory deprivation in the bad self are a reservoir of unrealized potentials that evolve from an absence of amplification, from a lack of opportunity, or due to conflict in the exercise of their functioning. These representations of sensory deprivation are elaborated into fantasies of emptiness. Deprivation is not an instinctual experience but refers to a deficit in sensory stimulation. It is important to distinguish it from the experience of frustration, which is associated with instinctual activity. Frustration is instinctually based, is represented in the bad self, and is the result of overstimulation. It reflects an effort to alleviate tension accumulated when there is a state of excess stimulation. The experience of frustration involves sensory activity, as opposed to its absence in deprivation. The fantasy of emptiness links to the representation of a depriving bad object and creates a union that functions especially well in defending against overstimulation. Repression proper, in its early phases, directs perceptual attention away from what is most threatening and focuses attention on what is least threatening. This defensive alignment is readily available for perceptual attention when there is an impending state of overstimulation.

The reactions to impingement represented in the bad self are elaborated into fantasies of fight, flight, and withdrawal. Reactions to impingement reflect the experience of moving away from an object and, hence, are less discriminatory. These representations of bad self-experience had been included in the boundary of unconscious mental activity prior to the development of an oedipal conflict. The formation of a new boundary for the unconscious system enables their participation in fostering the effectiveness of repression proper. The reactions to impingement, in and of themselves, reveal little of the nature of the impingement. They thus function to create a state of alertedness to respond defensively to any potentially noxious stimulus. The fantasies of fight, flight, and withdrawal are linked to the impressions of a bad impinging object, during the period of genital expansion, to provide a foundation for the effectiveness of castration anxiety. Instinctual experience involves intense engagement with an object and, as a result, is highly discriminatory. The advancing stages of psychosexual development are based upon the increasing discrimination of an enlarging range of body ego experiences. The impinging impressions of a bad object have been strongly affected by the instinctual impingements at the interior and are shaped by the particular stage in which they are registered. Oral impingements are represented as devouring, anal as sadistic, phallic as humiliating, and genital as castrating. Castration anxiety is structured during the period of phallic and genital expansion and incorporates the impinging representations of a castrating object. The union of reactions to impingements with the genitally determined impingements of an object enforces its prohibitive functions. The oedipal fantasies, which create a structured pathway for the integration of instinctual demands and a new boundary for the unconscious system, also motivate the formation of self- and object unions that foster more effective defensive activity.

The portal of entry of instinctual demand is represented as an instinctually overstimulating object and is elaborated into primal scene fantasies. During the period of genital expansion, these fantasies link to the representations of bad instinctual self-experience to structuralize an integrative pathway. The bad self and bad object are thus linked by two interrelated structures—one associated with defensive activity and forming a regulatory boundary for the unconscious system, and the other ensuring a continuous flow of instinctual demand. These instinctually based connections are the most advanced in the organization of the unconscious system, form a foundation that enables the shift from narcissism to object relatedness, and ensure stability and cohesiveness at the interior.

The instinctual impression of a bad object is the one facet of an object's influence that has no direct connection to an object in the external world. It is the mental impression of that dimension on the continuum of biophysiologic demand with the independent qualities of an object. The perception of an external object as instinctually overstimulating is determined by its influence. An external object can evoke its activity but not create its presence. The primal scene is a fantasy of an unseen object, instinctual in nature, mysterious, ominous, present but not present, overstimulating and resonating within self-experience but apart from it. It reflects the impact of the unseen dimensions on the continuum of biophysiologic demand. There are many individuals who have not perceived a primal scene in the external world and yet have represented it in the inner world. When the primal scene is perceived in the external world, its impact is a product of resonance with this fantasy elaboration.

The instinctual aspect of a bad object is located at the boundary of the unconscious system, and the other facets of a bad object's influence are accessible within the preconscious system. The representation of an impinging object is the product of impressions created by intrusive, unempathic interactions with an external object. The fantasies that are elaborated are shaped by the instinctual qualities of the impinging impact of biophysiologic demand and reflect the influence of the psychosexual phase of development in which they have formed. It is this aspect of a bad object's influence that is on a line of continuity of prohibitive experience, as optimally frustrating qualities shade into prohibitions and impingements. Selective identifications, initiated by the formation of the ego ideal, extend into identifications with an aggressor along this perceptual pathway. The demand for perceptual attention exerted by incestuous and primal scene fantasies, at the interior, activates defensive responses designed to support the effectiveness of repression proper. In addition, this demand motivates an acceleration of the selective identifications that strengthen the representations of good self-experience. When the intensity of instinctual activity is excessive or adaptive tasks weaken the self-representational system, identifications with an aggressor invoke more powerful prohibitions.

The object impressions of sensory deprivation, represented as a depriving object, are elaborated into fantasies of an object endowed with qualities that are deficient or needed and withheld. The fantasies readily link to the experiences of sensory deprivation, represented in the bad self, when compensatory idealizations are necessary as a defensive response. This aspect of an object's influence is also linked with fantasies of emptiness, when over-stimulation requires management.

The increase in instinctual activity associated with a genital consolidation requires a psychic organization in which the influences of an object are readily available for purposes of identification and for internal regulation. The genitally determined oedipal fantasies have structurally united the two systems of representation at the interior, by establishing a pathway of integration and a new boundary for the unconscious system. The organizing influence has extended throughout the personality as new defensive unions are effected, selective identifications are accelerated, and transitory identifications with an aggressor are invoked.

The New Structures Formed by the Oedipal Conflict

The formation of fixation points creates the perceptual stability necessary for an oedipal conflict to unfold and achieve a resolution in an orderly and sequential fashion. In health, a fixation point is formed on the projective arm of perception during the late oral period and fixated during the anal period. A second fixation point is formed on the introjective arm of perception furing the late anal period and fixated during the phallic period. In the neuroses, fixation points are formed and fixated in a delayed or premature fashion, maintain a defensive function, and serve as a background for the development of character pathology or the compromises of neurotic symptoms. In health, the oedipal conflict functions as a psychic organizer. In pathology, it emerges as a threat. The elaboration and resolution of an oedipal conflict is a crucial determining factor for the continuing integration of the demands of biophysiology and for the complex task of shifting from a narcissistic to an object-related orientation.

A fixation point is based on the memory traces of infantile experience and affects the perception of all stimuli. The varied stimuli emanating from the interior, and as a result of contact with the external world, are all given a similar meaning. Thus, in the presence of a fixation point, the degree of stability is increased, although the range of perceptual experience is narrowed. The formation of a fixation point on the introjective arm of perception has provided the degree of stability necessary for the structure of castration anxiety to consolidate. The resulting regulatory capacities and perceptual stability are sufficient for the genital fantasies of the oedipal conflict to flourish and to exert their function as a psychic organizer.

The representations of bad instinctual self-experience and of a bad instinctual object are structurally linked to each other and enable the shift from narcissism to object relatedness. In addition, the other aspects of bad self-experience and of a bad object's influence are united, through their fantasy elaborations, into new regulatory defensive constellations. The oedipal conflict thereby unites the self- and object representational systems in the realm of bad qualities of experience to form new structures for (1) a pathway for the integration of the drives, (2) a nonperceptual, but reactive, boundary for the unconscious system of mental activity, and (3) strengthening the effectiveness of repression proper in managing the overstimulating dimensions of genital instinctual activity.

The Pathway of Integration

The portal of entry of instinctual demand is represented as an overstimulating instinctual object. It is the impression of the dimension, on the continuum of biophysiological demand, with an intensity that could only be registered as having the qualities of an object. It has been so vigorously defended against, during the narcissistic phases of development, that the line of continuity with the representations of good and bad instinctual self-experiences is constantly interrupted. The evolution of the oedipal conflict, during the period of genital expansion, is manifested in the flourishing of primal scene fantasies. These fantasies, which reflect the increase in instinctual demand at its portal of entry, are linked to the representations of bad self-experience and structuralized.

The portal of entry of instinctual demand now has continuous access to representation within the self-system for the first time. The presence of an uninterrupted structured pathway facilitates the flow of instinctual demand, which is granted fuller expression through the formation of derivatives. The dimensions of instinctual demands, which have been represented as a facet of bad self-experience, are potentially accessible to inclusion within the realm of good self-experience. Selective identifications, motivated by the oedipal conflict, strengthen the self-system and diminish the need for defensive responses. Those elements of instinctual demands, which no longer require defense, have attained secondary autonomy and can serve as a boundary for an evolving system of conflict-free functioning. This final step in a completed pathway of instinctual integration takes place with the resolution of the oedipal conflict. Ultimately, a conflict-free system will function at the point of perceptual contact with the external world.

The ability to perceive an object as having independent objects of its own and to represent the body ego experience of that perception has evolved from the organizing function of the oedipal conflict. In the internal world, the significance of this perception is the capacity to represent the unseen dimension of the self with object qualities. This is the traumatic dimension on the continuum of biophysiological demand. The oedipal situation has created the means by which it can be represented and has organized a new structure that enables the broadening of perception. The movement of a continuous influx of instinctual demand along a structured pathway of integration makes it possible to heal the early splits in the self. These splits are variously referred to as the "basic fault" (Balint, 1968), or as "the psychotic sector of the personality" (Bion, 1968), and occupy the deepest layers of the id of the dynamic unconscious. In the external world, the significance of this perception is in the enhancement of self-expansion through object-related experiences.

The fixation points, which have formed to provide the stability for an object-related orientation to develop, then have to change. Alterations in the fixation points are essential in order to make the newly developed capacity for object relatedness a viable experience. The fixation point on the projective arm of perception must be maintained to provide the structural stability for the self-system to have ready access to the differentiated influences of an object and for the mechanisms of projection to function. These mechanisms are an integral part of the development of thought, language, the formation of derivatives, and the use of intellecutal activities. However, this fixation point must undergo a process of depersonification to gain some measure of independence from the original infantile narcissistic attachments upon which it is founded.

A fixation point on the introjective arm of perception is necessary for a transient period, as the genitally determined oedipal fantasies organize new mental structures. It then operates as an obstacle to the internalization of new experiences and must be gradually relinquished. The process of resolution of the oedipal conflict is initiated as it evolves and increases the degree of instinctual representation that does not require defense. The fixation point on the introjective arm of perception, which has been based on a recognition of the good self's bad instinctual qualities, is dissolved as these bad qualities are included within good self-experience. The stabilizing function of this fixation point is no longer necessary, and the introjective arm of perception is once again open to new stimuli with a broadened capacity for object-related perceptions.

A genital consolidation, reflected by the oedipal situation, has solidified the interrelationship between the self- and object systems of representation. Object constancy is anchored, and advancing levels of self-regulation are becoming functional. In conjunction with the establishment of a structured pathway of integration, there now exists within the personality a means for the continuing inclusion of biophysiologic demands without the fusion–merger experiences that were necessary in early development.

The New Boundary for the Unconscious System

During the narcissistic phases of development, the boundary of unconscious mental activity was maintained by the representations of impingements and the reactions to them. This union formed a reactive, but poorly discriminating, boundary that rigidly limited the degree to which greater intensities of instinctual demand could be included. Instinctual demand with an impinging impact was defensively excluded from representation, which interfered with the continuity of instinctual experience. This narcissistic boundary must be replaced as the genitally determined primal scene fantasies are establishing a structured pathway of integration.

During the evolution of the oedipal conflict, and the associated emergence of object-related perceptions, the representations of bad genital instinctual experience are elaborated into incestuous fantasies. These incestuous fantasies link to the representation of a bad instinctual object to form a new structure that is especially suited to function as a boundary for the unconscious system of mental activity. The two new structures, linked by the genital oedipal fantasies, involve the bad instinctual aspects of the self and object in a mutually interdependent relationship. One, the structured pathway of integration, reflects movement from the bad instinctual object to the bad instinctual self and is linked by the primal scene fantasy of the object. The other, the new boundary for the unconscious system, reflects movement from the bad instinctual self to the bad instinctual object and is linked by the incestuous fantasies of the self. This new boundary is reactive, nonperceptual, and has the capacity to evoke derivative expressions of unconscious mental activity. The shift to object-related perceptions is stabilized by this genitally determined boundary, and its defensive regulation has sufficient flexibility to elicit derivatives that represent the unseen dimensions of instinctual demand.

The New Defensive Unions

The formation of a new boundary for the unconscious system has made the remaining aspects of bad self-experience and of a bad object's influence available to form new defensive unions in the preconscious system. The increase in intensity of instinctual demand, associated with genital, object-related body ego experiences, requires the regulatory function of these new defensive alignments to maintain a continuous flow. The representations of an impinging object and of the reactions to impingements, linked during the narcissistic phases of development to form a boundary for unconscious mental activity, are now freed to participate in the structuralization of castration anxiety and to maintain a readiness to institute defense. The representation of sensory deprivation is elaborated into a fantasy of emptiness that, when linked to the impression of a depriving object, is especially effective in protecting against the effects of overstimulation. The representation of a depriving object is elaborated into withholding fantasies that link to the bad self-experiences of sensory deprivation. This union is at the foundation of compensatory idealizations and can serve as a perceptual focus when more threatening instinctual experiences are exerting a demand for attention. These unions are utilized to enforce the effectiveness of repression proper, which has gained dominance as the major defensive activity of the ego.

The Oedipal Conflict in Males and Females

The particular configuration of the oedipal conflict varies in each individual and is a different experience for boys and girls. The differences are based upon body ego experiences, genetic and biophysiologic makeups, the nature of the autonomous ego functions, and the particular characteristics of contact with the external world.

The early oral period of symbiosis is similar in males and females, although the attitude of the nurturing figure may have an effect upon the qualities responded to with empathic resonance. The emphasis is upon providing the phase-specific instinctual gratifications and amplification of autonomous ego functions that facilitate the building of psychic structure. The feminine attributes of the primary nurturing object and the feminine influence upon the background object of primary identification have a profound effect on both male and female developments. The feminine influence establishes a foundation for attachment to an object that exerts its effects upon all succeeding attachments, and upon interactions with the multiplicity of external objects that occur in the shadow of this primary attachment. This poses a difficult task, for the boy and girl, when confronted with the demands of a genital orientation. The emerging awareness of genital sensations in the primary attachment to the mothering figure has a different significance for each.

In the pregenital periods of psychosexual development, phase-specific instinctual gratifications depended upon the body ego experiences of an empathic interaction. These body ego experiences moved from those centering around orality, to anal experiences of mastery and control, to phallic narcissistic experiences of exhibitionism. Gratification was the consequence of an external object's empathic responsiveness, and the representation of the experience contributed to the structure formation that enabled a genital consolidation to take place. The infantile attachments, upon which this budding genital organization is founded, create conditions that obviate against instinctual gratification with an external object. Genitally determined interactions, at this level of psychic organization, lead to disappointment and narcissistic injury. The oedipal situation is one in which gratification takes place only in fantasy.

The Male Oedipal Constellation

The consolidation of the component instincts into a genital drive establishes the genital as the symbolic organ of connection to an object. A budding awareness of genital sexuality in the attachment to the primary maternal object is readily overstimulating and mobilizes the signaling, regulatory functions of castration anxiety. A threat to the integrity of the genitals or its symbolic derivatives is evoked, which serves as a powerful motive to accelerate the selective identifications that strengthen the self-system of representations. The clarity and distinctness of the prohibition serves as an effective restraint and signals for defensive responses that aid in the repression of primal scene and incestuous fantasies. The qualities of an object that are most admired are those that amplify masculine attributes. The resulting identifications aid in solidifying gender identity, foster the integration of instinctual demands, and provide a solution to the underlying oedipal conflict.

Incestuous and primal scene fantasies, reflecting the activity of the representations of bad instinctual self-experience and of the bad instinctual impressions of an object, present a heightened element of instinctual danger. During this period of new structure formation, there is a potential for instinctual overstimulation, which mobilizes the regulatory signaling functions of castration anxiety. Masculine identifications are accelerated, strengthening the self-system by a firmer connection to the influence of external reality, and mastery is achieved through the utilization of talents and skills. The ascending dominance of the reality principle encourages interactions that further enhance masculine identifications. This is abetted by an increasing mobility, maturation, and the ability to adapt to an expanding world of external objects. The external world offers enlarging opportunities for the symbolic and sublimated expression of instinctual wishes. Maturation and intellectual development foster the narcissistically gratifying experience of the mastery of tasks. This stands in opposition to the potential threat of failure, when behavior is motivated by oedipal fantasies.

The representations of good genital instinctual experience, and of a good genital object's influence, foster the view of a feminine object as the source of genital gratification. This must be delayed until the task of disengagement from infantile attachments to a primary object has been accomplished and a new independent object selected. The predominance of good self-experience that is evolving with the resolution of the oedipal conflict is associated with a greater ability to mobilize effective defensive responses. Repression proper is gradually able to be functional at the source of a stimulus, and the superego consolidates as an independent regulatory agency. The continuing process of integration is facilitated, which strengthens the experience of autonomy.

In the boy, a negative oedipal configuration is a reflection of pathology. The need to displace genital instinctual interest to the male figure requires the relinquishment of the genital as a symbolic organ of attachment and an emphasis on feminine identifications that is extreme. The perception of the male as a genital instinctual love object occurs as a consequence of an inordinate need for defense and creates a distortion in the development process. For the boy, the love object remains the same; it is the nature of the attachment that changes.

The Female Oedipal Constellation

The body ego experiences of genital exploration and the difficulty in differentiating body geographic areas (due to the proximity of genital and anal innervations) affect the girl's genital orientation. The conditions of genital instinctual gratification have been shaped by body ego experiences of genital exploration, and the awareness of genital sexuality in the primary attachment to a maternal figure is associated with an experience of disappointment. The maternal figure is seen as unable to provide the genital satisfactions that her body ego experiences demand. The structure of castration anxiety incorporates prohibitive impressions of an object that has been influenced by this experience. The primary maternal object is perceived as having been injured or damaged, to explain the disappointment, and castration anxiety is manifested in the threat of exposing similar damage to the self. The discovery of anatomical differences is often experienced as a narcissistic injury. Genital instinctual arousal is muted by the feeling of disappointment, so that the threat of overstimulation is not as great. The prohibitive regulatory and signaling function of castration anxiety is also not as pronounced, which diminishes the rapidity with which selective identifications are utilized as a solution to the oedipal conflict.

Genital instinctual expansion has engendered a more differentiated perception of the male attachments developing in the shadow of the primary attachment to a maternal figure. Disappointment in the mother intensifies the genital sexual awareness of, and interest in, the father. The rivalrous attitude that accompanies this genital interest, in combination with the disappointment already present, makes the process of feminine identification difficult. The motive for accelerating selective identifications that solidify gender identify, rather than being instigated by a threat of damage or injury (as in the boy), is based upon assuming a genital instinctual attitude toward the male figure. Thus, in the girl, the capacity to represent and integrate the instinctual demands of a consolidated genital drive is greater than in the boy. The establishment of a solid sense of sexual identity is more difficult for the girl, which is reflected in an emphasis upon phallic narcissism and in an extended period of oedipal conflict resolution. The negative oedipal situation is a developmental step in the girl, rather than an expression of pathology. The primary pregenital attachments to the maternal figure expand to include a genital instinctual aspect. It is experienced as a period of genital sexual awareness of, and attraction to, the mother. The feeling of disappointment leads to a displacement onto the father, who is then perceived as a genital sexual object. A motive is present to engage in those selective feminine identifications that strengthen the self-system and aid in consolidating a functional superego.

During the period of new structure formation, incestuous and primal scene fantasies are regulated by the structure of castration anxiety and the defensive reinforcement of repression proper that it signals. The girl is less in danger of instinctual overstimulation and more vulnerable to humiliation because the prohibitive function of castration anxiety is more modulated. The gradual resolution of the oedipal conflict is accompanied by the exercise of autonomous functions in the conflict-free sphere, available avenues for the sublimated expression of instinctual wishes, the assertion of feminine identifications, and mastery of adaptational tasks.

The pregenital phases of psychosexual development have involved a narcissistic overevaluation of experience. All aspects of perceptual contact have had meaning only in terms of how the self was enhanced by the object. With the development and resolution of an oedipal conflict, it is possible to enhance and strengthen the self through object-related experiences. The resolution of the oedipal conflict establishes a foundation that enables self-expansion to continue through involvement with new objects and new interests in the external world. The narcissistically determined structures are organized in a hierarchy to occupy the id of the dynamic unconscious, where they continue their function of representing the increasing quantities of the demands of biophysiology. In addition, they provide the depth of meaning to new perceptions that emphasize the uniqueness of an individual.

The Significance of Object-Related Perceptions

When cohesiveness is fully established and insured, perceptual experience reverberates throughout the entire personality. The manner in which stimuli are registered, as well as the meaning they are given, is determined by the structural composition of the varying systems of consciousness in which they are received. A stimulus may emanate from the continuum of biophysiological demand at the interior (the self with object qualities), or it may originate from the primary object in the external world (the object with self-qualities) or from a multiplicity of external perceptual contacts. The organizing influence of the oedipal conflict solidifies continuity, strengthens perceptual borders and areas of focused perceptual activity, and facilitates the formation of derivatives to express the unconscious meaning of experience. The borders of the projective and introjective arms of perception, the eye of consciousness and superego eye, and the new flexible, reactive boundary of the unconscious system all have an effect in determining meaning at different levels of organization. The psychological functions involved in establishing meaning operate under regulatory principles that vary in defined sectors of the personality. A stimulus registered in the id of the dynamic unconscious is governed by the pleasure principle, and its effects on the structures in the preconscious system are regulated by the grandiose self. The connection to the mental contents of the conscious system is governed by the reality principle and regulated by the ego ideal.

When the capacity for object-related perceptions is functional, external objects are seen as having unique characteristics and qualities that are separate and independent. These qualities can be more clearly identified and include their genital sexual aspects. Thus an external object can be seen as nurturing, as providing opportunities for the exercise of autonomy, control, and mastery, as reflecting acceptance of phallic achievements expressed through exhibitionism, and also as possessing genital sexual attributes. An object-related perception encompasses the recognition of an external object's having an independent genital sexual existence. In order to maintain this perception in a consistent fashion, much confidence in the stability of self-experience is necessary.

Confidence in self-stability is founded upon a number of interrelated conditions. The background object of primary identification and the representations of good self-experience have to be sufficiently structuralized at the interior, so that there is no longer a need for fusion–merger experiences. The differentiating and unifying structures of the grandiose self and ego ideal must be functional, to absorb and regulate the inevitable narcissistic injuries entailed in interactions with external objects. An uninterrupted, well-regulated, and structured pathway for the integration of instinctual demands is needed, to attain the secondary autonomy and sublimatory activities essential for healthy adaptation. Continuity of experience must be secured to foster the sense of identity and autonomy. Selective identifications, guided by a functioning superego, provide a source of strength that facilitates engagement with external objects, even when the potential is present for narcissistic injury. This pathway must be open and functional to diminish the need for narcissistically enhancing self-reflecting interactions.

The capacity for object-related perceptions is dependent upon, and an outgrowth of, the organizing influence of an oedipal conflict. Genitally determined primal scene fantasies have formed a structuralized linkage that enables the perception and integration of the unseen dimensions on the continuum of biophysiologic demand. The influx of instinctual demand, which had been potentially threatening and disruptive, now has a regulated pathway. The continuous flow of instinctual activity adds viability to self-experience and provides the motivating force for progressive thrusts toward self-expansion.

A genital object-related orientation is manifested in several ways. The recognition of genital sexuality, in the attachment to a primary object, is accompanied by the experience of increasing independence and differentiation. Genital sexuality is openly acknowledged, and clearly defined boundaries are established. The representations of good genital instinctual experience are elaborated into fantasies of desirable new objects. The fantasies are shaped by past and present experiences, curiosity, and intellectual mastery of concepts. They express the wish to become more fully separated, individuated, and differentiated from the primary object. The awareness of triadic relationships adds depth to an enlarging range of interpersonal involvements. The experience of personal uniqueness is amplified, as the thoughts, reactions, and responses that contain individual meaning are expressed. The sublimation of instinctual activity gives a strong impetus to the use of autonomous ego functions in the service of mastery, as the conflict-free sphere becomes a more dominant force in the personality.

The advanced level of psychic organization, at the foundation of object-related perceptions, provides a framework for ongoing developmental progression to take place on a new basis. During the narcissistic phases, it was based on being loved; with the shift to object-relatedness, it is based on being able to love. Ultimately, the infantile attachments to a primary object will occupy a place in the hierarchy of the id of the dynamic unconscious, as they are gradually replaced by the representations of attachments to new objects (from an object-related perspective).

Discussion

The mental contents that were the focus of A's attention revealed his expanding capacity to represent instinctual activity. The representation and elaboration in fantasy of anal, phallic, and now genital body ego experiences were abundantly present. The effects of early developmental traumata, upon the emerging anal-genital experiences, could be inferred. A's genital fantasies of reproduction, and anxiety concerning a genital attachment to a female, reflected the beginning evolution of an oedipal conflict. The fantasy of the therapist occupied with a woman, and separated from him, reflected a developing capacity to perceive an object as having independent objects. It appeared to reflect a shift that was taking place, from a narcissistic to an object-related orientation. The quality of his longing for a relationship with a girl gave some indication of the change, as it was always associated with an anxious awareness of the girl's involvement with others. These kinds of perceptions had been totally unavailable to him earlier. Up to this point, an object was only significant in relation to what it could bring to him. Now he showed a budding capacity to be enhanced through involvement with an object.

The extreme degree of conflict, associated with an object-related perception, was demonstrated in his enormous fear of females and in the idea of moving into dark and unknown territory. They both represented an unseen dimension with ominous, instinctual qualities. His association to the cave was possible, due to the emerging capacity to represent the unseen aspects of an experience. A was displaying the formation of a new structure, linked by primal scene fantasies, that was establishing a pathway of integration. Instinctual demand with the qualities of a bad instinctual object was gaining access to representation within the realm of bad instinctual self-experience. It could only be sustained with the support of the therapist's interpretive interventions. A could imagine looking into the darkness with the help of the guide's flashlight; that is, the therapist's interpretations and presence alleviated his anxiety enough so that he could perceive without its being an overwhelming threat. This metaphorical communication seemed to capture the essence of the structured pathway of integration that is at the foundation of object-related perceptions. The same theme was expressed in response to the therapist's closed door. A saw the closed door, imagined the therapist with an unseen instinctual object, and felt an upsurge of panic. This primal scene derivative is dependent upon the union of a bad instinctual impression of an object, through its primal scene fantasy, to the representation of a bad instinctual self-experience. The inordinate degree of anxiety, associated with this primal scene fantasy, is a function of the intensity of the conflict and the degree of pathology.

The formation of a new structure to function as a boundary for the unconscious system was indicated in the numerous fantasies of sexual union with an object. These derivatives, of incestuous fantasies, most frequently involved male figures. A's evolving oedipal constellation reflected the strong influence that anal experiences, and early experiences with mothering, were exerting upon this later genital expansion. A negative oedipal configuration was elaborated that operated as a protection from the enormous threat posed by perceiving the female as a genital instinctual object. There were many associations to sexual unions with males, which were accompanied by a minimum of anxiety and a high level of excitement. These incestuous fantasies were associated with defensive responses that were effective in supporting the repression of a more dangerous union with a female. Primal scene fantasies reflected a positive oedipal attachment and a structured pathway for instinctual integration. Incestuous fantasies reflected a negative oedipal attachment and a new boundary for the unconscious system.

The anxiety associated with primal scene fantasies, and to a lesser degree with incestuous fantasies, was a manifestation of the underlying structure of castration anxiety. This structure had consolidated the lines of continuity of instinctual and prohibitive experience and provided a regulatory and signaling function. A was deeply concerned with the integrity of his genitals, which had ascended as the symbolic organ of attachment to an object. The anxiety accompanying the threat of genital injury aided him in the regulation of increasing intensities of genital instinctual demand. A's oedipal constellation was inordinately conflicted. He longed for a genital attachment to a female, and though this was an experience fraught with danger, it gave expression to a progression toward establishing a positive oedipal attachment. A's derivative association to the danger of the dark cave, and the safety offered by the guide and his light producing function, indicated a capacity to achieve a resolution of the conflict. The potential for fixation in a negative oedipal configuration, and the degree of defensive distortion that it entailed, seemed to validate the concept of a negative oedipal conflict as a reflection of pathology.

The formation of new object-related structures provided a foundation that allowed the earlier profound splits in the self to be healed. It was noteworthy that the most threatening aspects of A's oedipal conflict were those representing a bad feminine object's influence. The bad genital instinctual impression of an object was represented as an overstimulating dangerous female, and the genital castrative, prohibitive influences of an object had feminine qualities. Males were represented as less threatening instinctual and prohibitive influences. This was in contrast to the fragmented representation of an object's influence that predominated initially. Objects with feminine qualities were depriving (The Big Pain), and those with male qualities were dangerously prohibitive (the Big Black Pops). This seemed to be a consequence of the effect of the therapeutic symbiosis upon the consolidation of self- and object entities. It also could be inferred that the earliest contact with a maternal figure had an impinging impact that could not be represented. Thus, as the capacity to represent the unseen dimensions of an experience was realized, it was colored by this early impression.

The patient, I, gave evidence of a negative oedipal constellation and of a movement toward displacing genital interest to the male. This step had created inordinate conflict and blocked her developmental progression. She developed a symptom, expressing the compromises that were effected, in regulating the conflict associated with genital instinctual activity. The negative oedipal position emerged as a developmental step that was maintained for defensive purposes. Her intense fear of a genital instinctual attachment to a male was implicitly manifested, early in the therapy, by the need to maintain a fixed perception of the therapist as a helping figure.

The therapeutic relationship intensified, and the patient became aware of openly incestuous dreams. She regarded them with an attitude of puzzlement and mild curiosity. These incestuous mental productions were accompanied by defensive responses reflecting the effectiveness of repression. This seemed consonant with the concept of incestuous fantasies representing the functional activity of a boundary for the unconscious system, structuralized by the oedipal conflict. The increasing intensity of instinctual demand was acting to mobilize the defensive functions of this new boundary.

The patient then began to experience body sensations of itching, and derivatively, demanded something from the therapist. The conscious demand was for the therapist to talk; the unconscious significance was the wish for a genital attachment. The therapist's interpretation linked these two facets of her experience together. *I* responded with representational imagery consonant with the concept of a structured pathway of integration. She giggled and then cried, as she thought of a joke that embodied the idea of genital union. She noticed the similarity between her itching, her symptom, and her genital arousal. In this context, she recalled the experience of perceiving the therapist's closed door. It had instigated a fantasy of an unseen sexual encounter. As she began to imagine the therapist with another figure behind the closed door, the mounting instinctual arousal and anxiety were so great that she had to exclude them from consciousness. The memory of this primal scene fantasy was associated with a freer flow of associative connections and greater access to the representations of self-experience. It appeared to be founded upon a structured linkage from the bad instinctual impressions of an object, via primal scene fantasies, to the representations of bad instinctual self-experience.

I's early development had become fixated during the oedipal period. The oedipal conflict had organized a new boundary for the unconscious system, manifested by incestuous fantasies, that was overdeveloped and reinforced the inordinate need for defense. The structured pathway of integration, manifested by primal scene fantasies, was heavily defended against and only intermittently functional.

The oedipal situation has had the effect of organizing a structural foundation that strengthens cohesiveness at the interior and of fostering the effectiveness of integrative processes at the periphery. The elaboration of an oedipal conflict prepares the way for a shift from a narcissistic orientation, and its resolution results in negotiating the step to an object-related perspective. A successful resolution is accompanied by a gradual realignment of the representations of infantile experience, to facilitate the dominance of a conflict-free sphere as the guiding force in the personality. These changes require the presence of an independently functioning agency, capable of internal regulation and of guidance in adaptive responses to the external world. The superego is consolidated to function as such an agency, operating harmoniously with the interests of the ego, in conjunction with the resolution of the oedipal conflict.

Perceptual contact with the external world can be registered in the conflict free-sphere and simultaneously can resonate throughout the personality. Similarly, a stimulus originating from the demands of biophysiology can be registered in the id of the dynamic unconscious, resonate throughout the personality, and ultimately be represented in the conflict-free sphere. The new boundary for the unconscious system is connected by the formation of derivatives in the focused perceptual activities of the superego eye in the preconscious system and the eye of consciousness in the conscious system. Unconscious perceptions evoke derivatives of healthy or pathological interactions and express the significance of external stimuli. Internal stimuli evoke derivatives of instinctual activity and express the distorting influence of unconscious wishes upon the immediacy of experience. A functional superego monitors the integration of instinctual activity and guides adaptive responses. It is thus essential that a connection be maintained to the infantile representations of experience that is free of their distorting influence. An understanding of superego development is an important background for distinguishing the differences between derivatives of unconscious perceptions and of instinctual activity. This distinction serves as a guideline for the therapist's participation in a therapeutic interaction. A containing, unconsciously empathic therapeutic environment, which does not stimulate the need for defensive, adaptive responses, is an essential condition to facilitate the expression of transference fantasy distortions.

CHAPTER 8

The Resolution of the Oedipal Conflict

The Consolidation of the Superego into an Independently Functioning Agency and the Process of Alteration in the Fixation Points

Introduction

Internal diaglogue is an an almost universal phenomenon that takes different forms and is given different names. Depending upon the circumstances and the internal makeup of the individual, it may be referred to as talking to oneself, praying, intrusive ideation, or as a hallucinatory experience. It involves an act of internal communication, with one inner entity engaged with another. There may be unity and harmony between these communicating entities; there may be conflict and opposition; or one may be split off from the other. This phenomenon appears to reflect the focused perceptual activity of the system ego (the eye of consciousness) engaged with the focused perceptual activity associated with the superego (the superego eye). The interrelationship between these two focused areas of perceptual activity, operating in different sectors of the personality, indicates the level of psychic organization that has been attained.

The superego is most frequently described as an independent agency within the ego or as a system of varied functions operating within the ego. The functions attributed to the superego are those that offer restraint, regulation, and guidance. These are qualities that reflect the influences of an object, and yet, for the superego to function as a system, it must be free of those influences. Webster defines a *system* as a set of facets, principles, and rules arranged in a regular, orderly form so as to show a logical plan linking the various parts. An *agency* is defined simply as an active force. These definitions emphasize that a system or agency does not exist until the various parts have been integrated into a unity. This is particularly important in relation to the functions of the superego.

From the very early phases of development, there are clearly observable indications of the presence of restraining and regulatory forces in the personality. These have often been presented as evidence that a functional superego is in existence, long before oedipal resolution is attained. Although this important observation has added much to the understanding of the early precursors of superego development, it becomes confusing when the precursors are portrayed as the system or agency of the superego. There is a significant difference between restraining and regulatory forces operating in isolation and those that operate in concert with each other that are linked to all other aspects of mental functioning. A system or agency of mental activity requires the presence of specific structures responsible for a given function, boundaries to contain them, and regulatory principles to govern their activity. It is necessary to differentiate the precursors of superego development from the superego itself and to define the processes by which these precursors consolidate to form a functional system. It is also essential to formulate the lines of development that have enabled the consolidated superego to maintain a functional connection to all other systems of mental activities. The superego has a conscious, preconscious, and unconscious dimension, includes a focused area of perceptual activity, and serves a regulatory and guiding function. A healthy, integrated, harmoniously functioning superego may make it difficult to delineate its separate facets, whereas in pathology the varied functions are more noticeable. However, a workable formulation should illuminate the manifestations of a given function in health and the effects of pathology upon that same function.

It has long been known that perception is a major function of the superego and that the superego's perceptual focus is linked to the function of self-observation. However, the function of self-observation and the perceptual function of the superego, though linked to each other, manifest differing qualities of perception. Perceptual activities in a conscious waking state and perceptual activities in the state of sleeping have similarities and differences that need to be explained. These differing qualities of perception are on a continuum with each other; this is demonstrated in examining the process by which a dream is remembered and then reported. It is also evident in the shifting qualities of perception that occur during the regressive experience of an analytic interaction. It is thus important to define the developmental line of these differing perceptual functions and the manner in which they are connected.

The relationship between wishful and realistic self-imagery has often been noted, though the process by which one is transformed into the other has not been fully understood. The emergence of the ego ideal as a facet of the superego has appeared to be involved in that transformation. In many instances, the varied functions of the superego are in opposition to each other and to the interests of the ego. This occurs when the oedipal conflict creates an inordinate need for defense, which interferes with its resolution. The transformation of wishful self-images to realistic self-images is then incomplete, and the ego ideal is not integrated into a smoothly functional superego. A fully consolidated superego only emerges as the conflict engendered by the oedipal situation is resolved. A need exists for further clarification of the role of the ego ideal in superego development that delineates the process by which harmony and integration is achieved.

Webster defines *independence* as a state that is not subject to the control, influence, or determination of others. Individuals who continue to rely upon external objects for internal regulation have not attained this developmental milestone. An integrated, harmoniously functioning superego, though independent, possesses qualities that are parallel with the parental attitudes of early development. Independence from these external influences is attained, in conjunction with the evolution of the superego from its early precursors, into a dominant, regulatory force within the personality. This agency has to possess an evocative resonance with all other agencies and systems within the mental organization of a given individual. These include the varied systems of consciousness, the id of the dynamic unconscious, the ego, the self- and object systems of representation, and the conflict-free sphere. There is an intimate interplay of forces within all of these mental agencies, with each being dependent upon the others for their effectiveness.

Unconscious, preconscious, and conscious mental activities are present on a continuum, with a set of boundaries and regulatory principles to define each area. The id, in its primitive form, reflects the transition from the realm of biophysiology to the realm of mental representation with a boundary of primal repression. The id is organized into a system, structured by the representations of advancing phases of narcissistic experience, which operates solely within the unconscious realm. The ego accomplishes the tasks of adaptation and of negotiating compromises between conflicting forces within the personality. It has access to all levels of consciousness. The systems of representations, based upon body ego experiences and object impressions, provide the mental background for all psychic functions. Finally, a conflict-free sphere is organizing that functions totally within the conscious system. The superego is the ultimate regulator of all mental activity and must be a part of, and differentiated from, these varied overlapping systems.

In this chapter, I will describe the precursors of the superego and the manner in which they consolidate into an integrated entity. I will also describe the interrelationship with all other systems and agencies operating within the personality.

Clinical Material

A's genital anxieties and preoccupations gradually receded. Thoughts concerned with a search for meaningful activities began to enter his mind. He was looking for activities that he liked and wanted to do and that would bring him more in contact with others. He wanted to belong to his peer group. He became absorbed with the idea of playing football. He watched it on TV and was fascinated by the intensity of physical contact. He developed a wealth of information about the various teams and players. His heroes were those who were most violent. He considered his own skills, fantasied being a player, entertained the idea of making it become real, and tried out for his high-school football team. In his fantasies he focused on the aspect of violence. The framework of a set of rules made it seem safer and more contained. It was reminiscent to the therapist of his earlier admiration of General Patton. *A* then described his awkward efforts to engage in the sport and of the limitations in his skills and coordination. He noted how impossible it was to carry the fantasied image of himself into his life. He became a member of the football team, although he rarely played. The following session took place immediately after *A* had talked of his ineptness, his lack of coordination, and the difficulties he encountered in becoming an active participant.

A began by evaluating his particular abilities. He decided to find an activity in which he could be more effective and selected track. In this sport, his determination could compensate for a deficiency in skills. He knew he could be relatively effective in running long distance. He could have the feeling of being both alone and a part of the group. He was by himself in running and yet did not feel isolated and on the sidelines. *A* then commented on the therapist's small stature, wondered how strong the therapist was, and whether he played football. He ruminated as to what would occur if he really let loose and attacked the therapist. Would the therapist be able to protect himself? Was he strong enough? The therapist stated that he thought *A* was remembering a time when the intensity of his aggression had been so overwhelming that it had spilled out into his diarrhea. He seemed to be wondering now whether the therapist's influence inside of him was sufficiently strong to contain his aggressive feelings. *A* became silent and then began to talk about the time coming closer to when he could be driving a car. The idea was exciting but also frightening. The prospect of being in charge of the car, starting, stopping, and steering it made him feel unchained. He also felt frightened. He imagined himself in heavy traffic, overwhelmed by the enormity of controlling the car, or on an expressway unable to master the speed. He fantasied difficult situations with other drivers looking at him or with cars speeding and getting in his way. He paused and stated with firmness and resolve, "If I am driving, I can also decide where to drive." He emphasized that it was his choice and that he could select places where he was capable of being in control. He could practice and improve his skills until he was better able to manage the car. Eventually, he would have sufficient control so as to not be overwhelmed.

J was a very bright and verbal 7-year-old boy. He was described as an ideal child during his first 6 years. He was neat, orderly, and conforming. He was the only male grandchild and "the apple of his grandparents' eyes." At the age of 6½, both grandparents died within a short period of time. J then appeared fearful, developed a series of bedtime rituals, and demanded that the family participate in them. He had to follow a set sequence, which, if interrupted, precipitated a temper tantrum or panic attack. His rituals were expanding, and the family, particularly his father, was feeling like a hostage to J's emotional well-being. In addition, he could not tolerate his parents' leaving for an evening and began to experience school difficulties for the first time. He could not complete easy reading assignments and would labor for hours on a simple task, tearing it up in frustration at the slightest mistake.

J began psychotherapy and found it difficult to talk. He sat immobilized in one place, was compliant, and appeared eager to please. He was curious about himself and puzzled about his reactions. In the early months, he described his symptoms and was puzzled as to why he felt so overwhelmed. His symptoms increased in severity, and he did worse in school, which was a profound blow to him. He became more hesitant, fearful, and unable to communicate verbally. He appeared frustrated by his inability to talk. He did not ask questions or seem to expect anything from the therapist. Slowly he revealed that he had been holding back important information from the therapist. However, he felt so guilty that he just could not say it. It had been on his mind from the first day. He finally mustered the courage and, with great difficulty, began to describe the deaths and funerals of his grandparents. Everyone around him had been devastated, whereas he had felt very little and pretended to be sad. The funerals were extremely exciting to him. There was activity and people that he found very stimulating. It was not until after these events that he began to be scared and guilty. The following session took place shortly after this revelation.

J began by talking rapidly and without hesitancy. All he could think about was numbers. He counted everything he saw. He had to end on a number that matched the number of members in his family. If he stopped at 3, he felt a disaster would occur; if he stopped at 5, he was terrified that he had separated himself from his family. He had to stop at 4 or 8 or 12. He was preoccupied with numbers and could not concentrate. He also could not read at school. He constantly anticipated that the next word would make him think of something awful. He was fearful of school and tests because he had to read. If someone asked him a question, that was okay; he just could not tolerate reading. At home he was becoming more and more fearful. He had to check the oven to see if the gas was off and then go back because he might have accidentally turned it on. In bed he had to be careful not to touch bare parts of his body. He had various rituals to cleanse himself and then had to be careful not to contaminate himself by touching. If he touched an exposed part, he had to wash his hands. His hands were red from washing so much. However, he had found a way to go to sleep. He did not know if he could tell it. *J* stopped, started, hesitated, and repeated his concern about saying it out loud. He paused and plunged on. ''I have this fantasy that I am the president. I've been afraid to tell you, cause if I say it out loud, the president will be assassinated.'' He had wanted to talk about it but felt fearful that the president would be shot. The therapist stated that he thought *J* was fearful of the sexual feelings that his symptoms were both hiding and expressing and was fearful that the therapist's recognition would shoot down the fantasy that protected him. *J* paused and began to talk about a friend he had invited to sleep over. They had become involved in sexual play by touching each other. It was extremely exciting, but he wondered if he was a homosexual. He fantasied himself growing up to be a politician, having this event in his childhood exposed, and then being publicly humiliated. The therapist commented on the guilt associated with his sexual arousal. *J* responded, ''Oh, I forgot to tell you. One of the things I worry about is the faucet dripping. By the way, do you have a faucet in here?'' *J*'s response made the therapist aware of his own feeling of excitement at the change in *J*'s ability to communicate. When *J* spoke of the leaking faucet, the therapist realized that *J* was sensing the therapist's excitement and that the memory of sexual play was a derivative expression of his experience with the therapist. The therapist remarked that *J* seemed to sense the therapist's excitement over the way he was talking and was fearful that the therapist was excited by his sexual fantasies and would be unable to contain it. *J* responded by describing the faucet that leaked in his house. He frequently went to check it and noticed his mother undressing in the bedroom as he passed. "Ooh, I almost forgot, my father asked me if he could talk to you." *J* went on to describe his father's anger at being enslaved by *J* and his anger that *J* controlled the house by controlling his mother. *J* then stated with relief that he knew the therapist would not talk to his father and that it felt good to be able to say no to his father with confidence.

The Structural Precursors of the Superego: Negotiating the Shift from Narcissism to Object Relatedness

Narcissism can be defined in a comprehensive fashion that includes its instinctual meaning, its significance for object relationships, as a state of the self, and as a phase in the development of the ego. Early experiences are totally narcissistic, until there is sufficient psychic structuralization for internal regulation to take place on a background of stability. Instinctually, an expanding range of narcissistic body ego experiences is reflected in the evolution of the component instincts. The impressions of an object's influence are determined exclusively by their narcissistic significance, reflected in the particular composition of the self- and object systems of representation, and manifested in interactions with the external world. A narcissistic focus of attention has been essential for negotiating the process of separation–individuation, which is reflected in the experience of a differentiated self. The amplification of autonomous ego functions has had a necessarily narcissistic focus. Continuing maturation and the exercise of unique individual skills enhances their viability and contribute to a narcissistically determined feeling of effectiveness.

The continuum of biophysiologic demand presents an ongoing stimulus, which is registered with differing qualities, reflecting the degrees of intensity (the self with object qualities). The external world presents stimuli with varying qualities, registered as object impressions, that have a containing, regulatory, restraining, and impinging influence. The interrelationship between the effects of these sources of stimulation results in an increasing capacity to represent instinctual activity and the formation of mental structures that establish a foundation for independent growth. The influences of an object are the precursors for organizing an intrapsychic agency, which is capable of monitoring the instinctual demands of the internal world and the adaptive demands of the external world. This agency, the superego, is gradually consolidated from its precursors into a functional entity as the pregenital narcissistic stages of development unfold.

In the earliest phases of development, body ego experiences are determined by the demands of orality. Instinctual gratification, restraint, containment, overstimulation, the exercise of autonomous ego functions, deprivations, and impingements are introjected to prepare for structure building by forming defined entities of mental representations. The process of separation-individuation is initiated, and the narcissistic instinctual focus changes to an emphasis upon anally determined experiences of control, mastery, and the advancement of autonomy. The recognition of separateness, as separation–individuation is negotiated, expands the boundaries of the self to attain a new level of psychic organization. Arms of perception are formed that connect the self- and object systems of representation, and a focused area of perceptual activity (the eye of consciousness) enables the organizing function of self-observation. A fixation point is established on the projective arm of perception, based on a recognition of the good object's bad anal qualities, which enable self-expansion to continue without the fusion–merger experiences that had previously been necessary. The introjective arm of perception remains open to the stimuli of the external world, relatively free of the effects of memory traces. Separateness is associated with the experience of vulnerability and helplessness. In conjunction with the availability of an object's influence and the stability provided by a point of fixation, a motive is present to form the first mental structure uniting and differentiating the systems of representations. This structure, the grandiose self, is based on participating in the fantasied omnipotence of an object and is a step toward consolidating the superego into an organized entity. The openness of the introjective arm of perception allows ongoing interactions, which facilitate instinctual expansion to be registered. A narcissistic interest in phallic body ego experience arises, at a time when adaptive capacities have been weakened from the involvement with fantasy embodied in the grandiose self. This motivates the formation of another new unifying and differentiating structure, designed to incorporate the influences of an object within self-experience. This structure, the ego ideal, is based on selective identifications and furthers superego consolidation. Cohesiveness is established, object constancy is anchored, and the component instincts are consolidated into a genital drive. The potential increase in instinctual activity cannot be contained and represented within a narcissistically structured personality, and a change in orientation is required. The formation of the ego ideal has directed perceptual attention into the self-system of representations, as phallic experience is at its height. The associated recognition of the good self's bad instinctual qualities establishes a fixation point on the introjective arm of perception. The resulting stability prepares the groundwork for a sequence of developmental events to occur, without the effects of responding to new external stimuli. The conditions are present that facilitate a more advanced level of psychic organization, which entails a shift from narcissism to object relatedness.

The primary motivating force for self-expansion and differentiation is the demand for perceptual attention exerted by the continuum of biophysiology. A narcissistic perspective has been necessary to negotiate separation–individuation and to establish a foundation for instinctual expansion to reach a genital focus. Once this has been attained, a potential state of trauma exists that can only be alleviated by the formation of new structures. Thus continued self-expansion depends upon the formation of an uninterrupted pathway for the integration of increasing intensities of instinctual demand and a regulatory force that is effective in guiding its expression. In order to accomplish this task, a new perception must evolve that is capable of including the previously unrepresentable dimensions of biophysiological demand. The representations of genital experience set in motion a sequence of events that culminate in a capacity for object-related perceptions—that is, a recognition of the object in the external world having independent unseen objects of its own and the ability to register the unseen, unintegrated dimensions on the continuum of bio-physiologic demand. The fixation point on the introjective arm of perception has stabilized cohesiveness sufficiently for genital fantasies to flourish and for new structures to form. The structure of castration anxiety is organized to serve a signaling, regulatory function and unites good and bad aspects of the self and object. It is a structure that reflects the instinctual self, striving for expression, in union with a prohibitive object, offering restraint and prohibition. Castration anxiety is capable of resonance throughout the personality and exerts an influence that ranges from the extremes of severe prohibition to gentle restraint. When good instinctual self-experience is involved, the firm gentle restraining influences of a good object are evoked. When bad instinctual self-experience is involved, the forceful prohibitive influence of a castrating impinging object are evoked. The structure and function of castration anxiety are intimately linked to, and an integral part of, the organizing superego. The conditions are present for the genital fantasies of the oedipal conflict to structuralize cohesiveness at the interior, by establishing a pathway of integration and a new boundary for the unconscious system. A foundation is organized for self-expansion to take place through object-related experiences and for a continuing influx of instinctual demand to be maintained.

The gradual resolution of the oedipal conflict is initiated with its onset, by accelerating the selective identifications that strengthens good self-experience. The resulting integration of bad instinctual self-experience is accompanied by a dissolution of the fixation point on the introjective arm of perception, which allows new object-related experiences to be registered. The structural precursors of the superego are integrated into a functional entity in proportion to the degree of resolution that is attained. The borders of the grandiose self and ego ideal are organized into an internal area of perceptual functioning, which I have refered to as the "superego eye." The grandiose self remains as a narcissistic structure that functions to register the perceptions of mental contents in the deeply preconscious system and to regulate the effects of unconscious mental activity. The ego ideal slowly changes from a narcissistic to an object-related structure as selective identifications, involved in the resolution of the oedipal conflict, become object related. The ego ideal registers the perception of mental contents in the transition from the preconscious to conscious systems and regulates conscious mental activity. Repression proper, which has emerged as the primary defense of the ego, is guided by the signaling function of castration anxiety. In its initial phases, perceptual attention can be directed toward less threatening defensive alignments, and away from more threatening instinctual derivatives. Ultimately, as the regulatory influences of an object are harmonious with the interests of the ego, repression proper can function effectively at the source of instinctual activity.

The Polarization of Superego Functions: Splits in the Superego

The intrapsychic events, leading up to the elaboration of an oedipal conflict, have all involved a gradual process of organizing the influences of an object into a functional entity—the superego. With the onset of cohesiveness, these object influences have enabled expanding degrees of self-regulation. In sequence, a series of developmental steps establishes the necessary conditions for the superego to emerge as an effective guiding and regulatory agency. A fixation point is formed on the projective arm of perception that binds the line of continuity of prohibitive experience and furthers differentiation. The grandiose self provides a pathway by which fantasied influences of an object can compensate for vulnerabilities. The ego ideal provides a pathway for the impressions of an object to be included within self-experience to strengthen weaknesses and deficiencies. A fixation point is formed on the introjective arm of perception for stability, which supports the consolidation of the component instincts into a genital drive. Castration anxiety pulls all aspects of mental representation into closer apposition, by uniting the lines of continuity of prohibitive and instinctual experiences. The genital fantasies of the oedipal conflict then flourish, new structures are formed, and the superego gains dominance as an independently functioning agency.

In the early stages of superego consolidation, a polarization of functions is proportional to the degree of resolution of the oedipal conflict. Experiences of genital instinctual overstimulation exert a demand for perceptual attention that must be effectively regulated and defended against to facilitate the shift to object relatedness. Prohibitive superego functions are elicited at the source of the stimulation, and idealizing superego functions are activated at a separate locale, in order to support the ego in directing perceptual attention away from what is most threatening and toward what is least threatening. Thus prohibitive influences are present at the pole where self-experiences have been represented, and compensatory idealizations occur at the pole where the impressions of an object have been represented. This is a manifestation of repression proper, which has replaced splitting as the primary defense of the ego. The earlier translocations of perceptions, which have been healed, are now reflected in a cohesive state as splits in the superego. A harmonious balance between these polarized functions is achieved as the oedipal conflict is resolved and as the influences of an object are in accord with the interests of the ego. It is then possible for defensive responses to regulate instinctual activity on a continuous pathway toward integration, and perceptual attention can be maintained at the source of a stimulus.

The portal of entry of instinctual demand is represented as an overstimulating instinctual object. During the period of oedipal organization, the elaboration of genital primal scene fantasies are structurally linked to the experiences of genital overstimulation represented in the self-system. This new structure performs several interrelated functions. It insures cohesiveness at the interior, provides the foundation for an object-related perception, and creates a pathway that enables the unseen dimensions of instinctual demand to gain access to representation within self-experience. The experiences of genital overstimulation in the self-system, are on a line of continuity with the representations of good instinctual self-experience and exert a demand for perceptual attention that must be modulated to support the effectiveness of their repression. The prohibitive influences of an object are potentially available to accomplish this task.

In the early symbiotic period, primitive identifications took place in a state of lack of differentiation. The empathic responsiveness of an external object amplified the use of autonomous functions, and the object's influence was thus an integral part of self-experience. In a more advanced state of differentiation, identifications occur within the internal world. The autonomous functions are elaborated into fantasies that link to qualities of an object's influence that are needed and hence admired. This process of selective identification has been involved in forming the ego ideal and is a more advanced expression of including the influences of an object within self-experience. The line of continuity of prohibitive experience, which represents the impressions of a good restraining object and shades into the impressions of a bad impinging and prohibitive object, makes the prohibitive influences of an object available for purposes of identification. This process, of identification with an aggressor (a prohibitive object's influence), establishes the prohibitive function of the superego at the pole of self-experience.

The resolution of the oedipal conflict is also attained through selective identification that, in strengthening the self-system, expand the degree to which instinctual activity can be included without the need for defense. The impulsion of instinctual demand moves from its portal of entry to representation within bad instinctual self-experience, to inclusion as a facet of good self-experience. The end result is an established and regulated pathway of integration.

The Integration of Superego Functions: The Healing of Superego Splits

The self with object qualities operates as a continuous source of instinctual demand, with an unperceived dimension that is now capable of representation. This is equivalent to the experience of an external object's having independent objects that are reacted to though they cannot be directly perceived. Prior to the shift from narcissism to object relatedness, this perception was potentially too traumatic. An instinctual pathway of integration is structured that moves from the unconscious system at the interior to the conflict-free sphere in the conscious system at the periphery. The dimensions of instinctual demands, which have been unintegratable, now motivate and participate in continuing self-expansion. This instinctual pathway requires the presence of a monitoring agency within the personality, and the superego consolidates from its precursors to serve that function. The influences of an object are organized into a structured entity that maintains an evocative connection to all aspects of mental representation, provides regulation for instinctual activity, and guides adaptive responses to the external world.

The regulatory function of the superego increases in its efficiency as the oedipal conflict is resolved through selective identifications. The process of including a good object's influence within good self-experience strengthens the self-system and diminishes the need for severe prohibitions and compensatory idealizations. Instinctual activity, which previously was overstimulating, can then be represented without requiring defense. The availability of modulated defensive responses enables the ability to regulate an ongoing process of integration, which insures a continuous flow of instinctual activity throughout the entire personality. The effectiveness of repression proper is more firmly established, and perceptual attention can remain at the source of a stimulus. The splits in the superego are healed, as the polarization of functions is alleviated.

The oedipal conflict has been directly involved in attaining a new level of psychic organization, by structuring the foundation for a change in perceptual perspective. The shift from a narcissistic to an object-related orientation is essential for self-expansion to continue when the component instincts have consolidated into a genital drive. The oedipal conflict also exerts an organizing influence upon all other facets of the personality. A new boundary for the unconscious system and a structured pathway of instinctual integration increase the capacity for instinctual representation. The intrapsychic conflict, engendered by the flourishing genital oedipal fantasies, accelerates the selective identifications essential for its resolution. This motivates, and is an integral part of, the organization and integration of object influences into a superego that functions as an independent regulatory and guiding agency. It regulates instinctual demands emanating from the interior, adaptive responses to external stimulation, and guides in the selection of external objects and sublimatory activities.

Selective identifications with the influence of a good object enhance the inclusion of instinctual demand within good self-experience. Instinctual activity, traversing the pathway of integration, attains secondary autonomy and access to the conflict-free sphere. The conflict-free sphere is an extension of the autonomous ego functions that is organizing as a system, at the point of perceptual contact with the external world. The superego, which is emerging as a dominant force within the personality, must maintain an intimate connection to this developing system to ensure that its functions are in harmony with the interests of the ego. Boundaries, for this area of conflict-free mental activity, are forming in conjunction with the resolution of the oedipal conflict. The inner surface is composed of the representations of instinctual demands that have attained secondary autonomy. An outer surface will evolve, which is composed of the representations of new empathic, object-related interactions that are free of conflict. Fusion–merger experiences, resulting from empathic contact with an external object during the early symbiotic period, take their place along with the other representations of narcissistic experience in the id of the dynamic unconscious.

With the establishment of a genitally determined object-related psychic organization, the tripartite structures of id, ego, and superego are clearly defined. The superego is integrated as a functional agency, with perceptual boundaries maintaining an evocative connection to all facets of the personality. The ego remains as the primary mediator of adaptive responses and is the source of executive, synthetic, defensive, and autonomous functions. The id is composed of a hierarchy of narcissistic mental representations that are organized to utilize instinctual energies with varying degrees of neutralization. These narcissistic structures are available for a variety of functions. They may be regressively and defensively invoked under excessively stressful conditions. They provide the underlying mental representations, necessary to make use of fluctuating degrees of neutralized instinctual energy, that give depth, richness, and meaning to new perceptual experiences. They are essential as a background for the momentary, transient regressions in the service of the ego involved in play and in empathic communication with others. Empathic communication requires an object-related orientation and enhances self-expansion.

The demands of biophysiology are registered within the id of the dynamic unconscious and gain advancing levels of neutralization. The representations of narcissistic experiences that are activated reflect the developmental history of the individual and initiate the process of integration. The most advanced expression of instinctual demand within the unconscious system is its portal of entry, which is represented as a genitally overstimulating object. The primal scene fantasies that are elaborated have been structurally linked to self-experiences of overstimulation, as the process of integration continues. The final step of instinctual integration occurs as it is included within good self-experience, where it participates in the changes in the fixation points.

Changes in the Fixation Points with Resolution of the Oedipal Conflict

The oedipal conflict has been elaborated in fantasy, linkages at the interior have been structured to insure cohesiveness, object-related perceptions have been made possible, a pathway for the integration of a continuing influx of instinctual demand has been created, and the shift from narcissism to object relatedness has been negotiated. The fixation points, which have been based upon a narcissistic infantile attachment and upon narcissistic phallic instinctual experience, must change for self-expansion to continue. A fixation point on the projective arm of perception must be sustained to anchor object constancy and must provide a background on which projective mechanisms can operate. However, an alteration is necessary to obviate the distorting effect of a narcissistic attachment to an object. A fixation point on the introjective arm of perception was essential during the period of genital consolidation and oedipal organization. There was then sufficient stability for the genital oedipal fantasies to flourish and for new object-related structures to form. When these structures are firmly established, this fixation point becomes an obstacle to the introjection of new stimuli and has to be gradually relinquished. Thus the fixation points undergo a transition to enable the stimuli of new object-related experiences to be registered and represented. The memory traces of their original composition recede to occupy a place in the organization of the id of the dynamic unconscious.

The passing of the oedipal conflict refers to the new level of psychic organization that is established with its resolution.. A framework is then present for object-related experiences to enhance a continuing process of self-expansion. The resolution of the oedipal conflict and the modifications and changes in the fixation points occupy the latency period of development.

The Fixation Point on the Projective Arm of Perception: The Process of Depersonification

The fixation point on the projective arm of perception was established with the recognition of the good object's bad qualities. It occurred during the anal phase, was based on a perception of the line of continuity of prohibitive experience, and reflects the attachment to an optimally frustrating object that can become prohibitive and anally sadistic. This fixation point served an important differentiating and stabilizing function. It allowed empathic interactions to be introjected and represented, without the loss of differentiation involved in experiences of fusion and merger. It also enabled cohesiveness to be furthered by forming the structures of the grandiose self and ego ideal, which united and differentiated the self- and object systems of representation at the periphery.

Negotiating the shift from narcissism to object relatedness ensures cohesiveness at the interior by forming a structured pathway of integration and a new boundary for the unconscious system. The fixation point on the projective arm of perception can expand its area of functioning beyond the original task of stabilizing cohesiveness because the necessity of this function has diminished. It must still be retained to support object constancy and the mechanisms of projection that are involved in thought, language, symbolization, and the expression of derivatives. This fixation point, which has been founded on a narcissistic attachment to an object, plays a role in determining the unique, individual meaning of a new stimulus. Unless it undergoes an alteration that can be adapted to an object-related orientation, that narcissistic influence will continue to exert an effect. It is thus important, for continuing growth, that this fixation point expand and include the representation of object-related attachments.

The negotiation of separation–individuation culminated in the recognition of a separate good object's influence. The intrapsychic manifestation was in the expansion of self-boundaries to create two arms of perception and a focused area of perceptual activity (the eye of consciousness). In this early narcissistic stage, the impressions of a good object were evocative of fusion–merger experiences, and the perception of a separate good object was difficult to sustain. The fixation point on the projective arm of perception stabilized the differentiated impressions of a good object, by the effects of perceiving its bad qualities. The conflict-free sphere, which is organizing at the periphery, contains the representations of empathic object-related interactions. They reflect the impressions of a good object that have been perceived and registered without endangering separateness. These memory traces are at the foundation of symbolic productions, ideational content, interests, and beliefs that are elaborated in the conflict-free sphere. Mental contents, representative of empathic interactions, are thereby depersonified. The fixation point on the projective arm of perception, which was initiated with the awareness of a separate good object's influence, resonates with the depersonified mental contents having a similar basis. The evocative connection, registered by the eye of consciousness, extends the original fixation point into the realm of the conscious system. This process of depersonification links object-related mental productions to the fixation point on the projective arm of perception, which lessens the effect of its infantile attachment and expands its area of functioning. The perceptual pathway, from the conflict-free sphere to the projective arm of perception, enables the process of depersonification to increasingly expand the stabilized foundation upon which conscious mental activities can proliferate.

The Fixation Point on the Introjective Arm of Perception: The Process of Integration

Concurrently, change is taking place in the fixation point on the introjective arm of perception. This fixation point was formed by the recognition of the good self's bad instinctual qualities. It provided the necessary stability for the oedipal conflict to exert its organizing influence. Selective identifications, involved in the resolution of the oedipal conflict, have strengthened the capacity for instinctual representation. Genital instinctual experience, which was overstimulating and required defense, can then attain secondary autonomy and be included within good self-experience. This final step in the integration of instinctual demand takes place along the line of continuity of instinctual experience, which has determined the composition of the fixation point. Thus the integration of instinctual activity is accomplished by a dissolution of the fixed perception that it created.

The resolution of the oedipal conflict is associated with the consolidation of the superego into a functional regulatory agency, which assures continuity of experience within the personality. Repression proper is gradually more effective as superego splits are healed and as instinctual activity can be defended against at its source. Cohesiveness is secured by the formation of new object-related structures at the interior. The original stabilizing function of the fixation point on the introjective arm of perception is no longer necessary and, to the extent that it remains, interferes with the introjection of new object-related experiences. The fixation point is slowly dissolved and relinquished while a system of conflict-free functions is organizing at the periphery, and stimuli are received relatively free of the effects of memory traces. New experiences are once again possible and perceived from an object-related orientation.

The introjective and projective arms of perception provide a pathway for stimuli to resonate throughout the personality, which is now cohesive and differentiated. The processes of instinctual integration and sublimation, occurring along the introjective arm of perception, delay incoming stimuli sufficiently to enable selective perceptual attention. The ongoing process of depersonification, on the projective arm of perception, creates the necessary delay for these incoming stimuli to be simultaneously registered in the conscious system as immediate perceptions within the conflict-free sphere and to resonate throughout the personality, activating all levels of perception. A given stimulus can thus attain the depth and richness of meaning that the individual's developmental experience has made possible. The intensity or nature of a stimulus determines the degree of delay that is necessary. A stimulus of great intensity over a short period of time may evoke only the more regressive areas of focused perceptual activity in the deeper layers of the personality and be traumatic.

The changes in the fixation points, expanding contact with varied objects in the external world, and an increasing influx of instinctual demand result in a proliferation of fantasy and an intensification of unconscious mental activity. Instinctual derivatives and derivatives of unconscious perceptions are more abundant, and symbolized mental contents accumulate within the conflict-free sphere. The process of depersonification is increasingly active, as symbolized expressions of a good object's influence are perceptually engaged by the eye of consciousness and connected to the expanding fixation point on the projective arm of perception. The fixation point on the introjective arm of perception has been gradually integrated and relinquished, so that new object-related perceptions, relatively free of memory, can be experienced.

The Relationship of the Consolidated Superego to Its Structural Precursors and the Functional Systems of Representation

The superego does not emerge as a functional and independent agency until the process of resolution of the oedipal conflict has begun. The various structured unions of self-experience and an object's influence that eventually comprise the superego are its genetic precursors. The sequence of events, in which the grandiose self, ego ideal, and castration anxiety develop, are all steps leading up to the organization of a separate independent structure. There is a point when these precursors have consolidated and achieved a sufficient level of integration to be called a superego. That point occurs when body ego experiences are registered in response to an unseen object. It reflects the ability to recognize the object as having independent objects of its own and to include the unseen dimensions on the continuum of biophysiologic demand within the realm of representation and regulation. In the absence of this capacity for object-related perceptions, a need remains for external objects to provide regulation. Individuals, who have not developed that capacity, are in a constant state of potential trauma and in need of restraining and defense reinforcing interactions in order to feel regulated. Harsh and punitive prohibitive responses to instinctual activity may be an indication of developing pathology, as superego precursors are overemphasized in the effort to attain self-regulation.

The perception of an external object, having an unseen independent instinctual life, is based upon the body ego experience of perceptual contact with the demands of biophysiology. For this reason, it does not require two parental figures in the external world to develop and elaborate an oedipal conflict. The conflict involves the fantasies that are elaborated from self-experiences of genital overstimulation and from the impression of a genitally overstimulating object. This latter impression does not result from contact with an external object but reflects the potentially traumatic dimension on the continuum of biophysiologic demand.

One essential aspect for attaining a level of psychic organization, in which an oedipal situation can evolve, has involved the inclusion of an object's influence within self-experience. With advances in differentiation, this process of identification becomes increasingly selective. The body ego experience of contact with the intrauterine environment, represented as the background object of primary identification, is the most primitive form of including an object's influence and is the foundation for all processes of identification. An individual can only identify with those influences of an object that are consonant with some aspect of self-experience. During the symbiotic period, an external object's empathic responses resonate with, amplify, or evoke self-experience. In this primitive state of lack of differentiation a stimulus that is outside of the self is represented and included within the self. When separation–individuation is negotiated, identifications can take place with the representations of an object's influence and be selective. Wishful images of self-experience are linked to the represented qualities of an object that match these fantasies of the self's potentials. Later, this process of selective identification is involved in the resolution of the oedipal conflict and the consolidation of the superego into an independent agency. The complex processes of identification, though on a developmental continuum with the more primitive forms, are different in their effects and manifestations. Similarly, the superego, as an independently functioning agency, is different than its genetic precursors.

The Grandiose Self

This is the first mental structure formed that unites and differentiates the system of self-experiences with the system composed of an object's influences. It is thus the onset of organizing the varied forces, developing in the personality, that can serve the purpose of self-regulation and guidance. These forces can be described as superego nuclei and their structuralization as superego precursors. The grandiose self is an instinctual structure, and the underlying motive for its formation is the experience of vulnerability associated with separateness. At this juncture, cohesiveness is extremely unstable, and it requires the power of an instinctual movement toward engagement with an object to effect the linkage. The good anal instinctual experiences of mastery and control are linked to the representation of an optimally gratifying object by its fantasy of omnipotence. The perceptual functions that are utilized in this search for a good object's influence are incorporated in the resulting structure and will ultimately serve as a focused area of internally directed perceptual activity. This superego precursor, based on participation in the fantasy of an object's omnipotence, is particularly suited to regulate mental contents operating under the pleasure principle and affected by primary process activity. It also solidifies cohesiveness, to the extent necessary, for selective identifications to be affected.

The Structure of the Ego Ideal

The formation of the grandiose self has balanced the experience of vulnerability but created an imbalance between instinctual experiences not requiring defense and those that are overstimulating. Adaptive and restraining functions within the self-system are weakened, which motivates a search for the qualities of an object that can be included within self-experience to strengthen it and reestablish a balance. This process of selective identification is a further step in the organization of the superego and forms the structure of the ego ideal. The weakened autonomous ego functions, represented as a facet of good self-experience, are elaborated into fantasies of potentials that are linked to admired qualities represented in the object. The perceptual functions that are utilized in the search are incorporated in the resulting structure and will ultimately serve as a focused area of outwardly directed perceptual activity. This superego precursor, based upon selective identification, is well adapted to regulate mental contents operating under the reality principle and affected by secondary-process activity. The combined areas of perceptual activity associated with the grandiose self and ego ideal form an internal focus of perception that I have referred to as the "superego eye." It is directed inward to perceive the contents in transition from the unconscious to preconscious systems, and outward to perceive the contents in transition from the preconscious to conscious systems. The ego ideal becomes more predominant with the emergence of the oedipal conflict because it provides the pathway for its resolution.

Castration Anxiety: The Lines of Continuity of Experience

The self- and object systems of representation have developed at opposite poles within the boundaries of the self. Each system has formed well-defined entitites, which have become localized, with good qualities of experience at the periphery and bad qualities at the interior. Although the body ego experiences that do not require defense are separate from those that require defense in the self-system and although the object impressions that do not elicit defense are separate from those that elicit a defensive response in the object system, there are lines of continuity of experience that maintain a connection between them. These reflect the impact of stimuli that are on a continuum but are represented differently as the quality of the stimulus changes.

Instinctual experience is on a line of continuity that moves from the interior to the periphery. It results from perceptual contact with the continuum of biophysiological demand, which is represented as having differing qualities as the intensity increases. The dimension not requiring defense is represented within good self-experience, shades into bad self-experience as it reaches overstimulating proportions, and extends to the impression of an overstimulating instinctual object when the intensity is to a potentially traumatic degree. During the pregenital narcissistic stages of development, this latter aspect is readily disrupted due to its traumatic impact and interferes with a continuity of experience. Prohibitive experience is on a line of continuity that moves from the periphery to the interior. It results from perceptual contact with the restraining influences of an external object, which extends from qualities of optimal frustration, represented in the good object, and shades into the prohibitive and impinging impressions of a bad object. The impingements mobilize defensive reactions within bad self-experience, which forms a rigid boundary for unconscious mental activity in a narcissistic organization.

A fixation point on the projective arm of perception connects the two systems of representations to initiate cohesiveness and anchor object constancy; this fosters a continuity of experience. The grandiose self and ego ideal solidify cohesiveness at the periphery and strengthen the bonds of continuity. However, it is not until the original lines of continuity of experience are structurally united that it can be fully assured. This is initiated, as the component instincts consolidate into a genital drive, with the structuralization of castration anxiety. This superego precursor maintains an evocation connection to all aspects of mental representation and is esential for regulating the new object-related structures that are organized by the oedipal conflict.

The affect of anxiety is present at every phase of development, and its nature is defined by the representations of the experiences upon which it is based. Castration anxiety is manifested during the period of phallic and genital instinctual expansion and is based upon a structural linkage of the lines of continuity of instinctual and prohibitive experience. This structure includes genitally determined good and bad instinctual self-experiences and the good and bad restraining, prohibitive, and impinging impressions of an object. It serves the unique function of signaling the need for defensive activity and provides the regulatory influence necessary for the oedipal conflict to flourish. The genital fantasies of the oedipal conflict firmly link the self- and object systems of representations at the interior, which ensures cohesiveness and continuity of experience within the personality. Primal scene fantasies reflect the linkage of the portal of entry of instinctual demand to the self-experiences of genital overstimulation, which structures the line of continuity of instinctual experience. A pathway of integration for the continuous influx of instinctual demand is then available. Incestuous fantasies reflect the linkage of bad genital instinctual experiences to the highly defended impression of an overstimulating instinctual object, which structures a new, more flexible boundary for the unconscious system. This genitally determined boundary enables the hierarchy of narcissistic representations to be organized into the id of the dynamic unconscious. The structured linkages of bad instinctual qualities of experience at the interior facilitate the union of other bad qualities of experience that function well as a response to the threat of overstimulation. The fantasy of emptiness elaborated from the experience of sensory deprivation linked to the impression of a depriving object and the fantasy of a withholding object linked to the experience of sensory deprivation are readily called to attention by the signaling function of castration anxiety. This defensive activity of repression proper is a manifestation of the increasing consolidation of superego precursors into a functional unit.

The Emergence of Repression Proper as the Major Ego Defense

In the early stages of development, the mechanism of splitting was the major defense available to a primitively organized ego. These splits in the ego were the result of a translocation of perception, in which a stimulus occurring in one locale was perceived in another. It enabled the formation and buildup of defined entitites of self-experience and allowed them to be represented where they were most needed. Good self-experience was consolidated at the interior to balance the disruptive effect of biophysiologic demand, and bad self-experience was consolidated at the periphery to balance the lack of differentiation in a symbiosis. The activity of splitting served a differentiating function, a defensive function, and provided a way to represent experiences of overstimulation.

Repression proper is initiated with the onset of cohesiveness and becomes the dominant defensive activity with the structuralization of castration anxiety. Initially, repression proper depends upon a similar process of splitting, in that perceptual attention is directed away from the source of stimulation. However, in this later phase of development, cohesiveness has been established, and the turning away of perception is not a translocation. A translocation involves a discontinuity of experience, and though perceptual attention is directed away from the source of a stimulus, there is resonance throughout the personality. The manner in which the stimulus is perceived, as it resonates, is determined by the focused areas of perceptual activities that form boundaries for the various systems of consciousness. Repression proper becomes more effective as the oedipal conflict is resolved. It is then no longer necessary to direct perceptual attention away from the source of stimulation, which reflects the integration of previously polarized superego functions and a healing of superego splits. Instinctual activity, in the process of integration, still requires countercathectic, repressive, and defensive regulation. However, these defensive responses are evoked at the site of the stimulus.

The Functional Systems of Representation

With the shift from narcissism to object relatedness, a genitally determined psychic organization predominates in the conscious and preconscious systems and is manifested at the boundary of the unconscious system. The pregenital narcissistic representations of self-experience and of an object's influence that require or elicit defense, and of undifferentiated experiences not requiring defense, are encompassed within the boundary of the unconscious system. Differentiated pregenital representations of good self-experience and of a good object's influence remain within the conscious system where they enable sublimatory activities and transient regressions in the service of the ego. When continuity of experience is secured within the personality, the structuralization of castration anxiety and its inclusion within a consolidated superego maintain a link of superego regulation to all aspects of instinctual experience. The composition of the functional systems of representation determine the pathway of integration, from its initiation in the id of the dynamic unconscious to attaining secondary autonomy; the formation of derivatives, expressing instinctual activity and the activity of unconscious perceptions; ideational and symbolic productions; and the advancing stages in the integration and organization of the superego.

The Good Self

Good selves are the representations of phase-specific instinctual gratification, of the activity of autonomous ego functions, of the background object of primary identification, and they include their fantasy elaborations. Complex nuances of discrimination evolve only in the representations of instinctual experience because instinctual activity motivates intense engagement with an object. Self-experiences that do not require defense are incorporated into the entity of a good self.

Initially, good instinctual self-experiences are based upon oral gratifications and elaborated into fantasies of total satiation. It is only the later phases of orality that remain because experiences of fusion and merger are incompatible with the level of differentiation and have receded into the deeper layers of the unconscious system. Instinctual expansion continues into the anal period as body ego experiences of control, mastery, and autonomy are represented and elaborated into fantasies of omnipotence. The grandiose self is formed during this period, and the structured linkage with the fantasy of an omnipotent object continues to aid in absorbing narcissistic injuries. Phallic body ego experiences of exhibitionism are elaborated into fantasies that include an audience, which reflects the very beginnings of movement away from a totally narcissistic perspective. The consolidation of these narcissistically determined component instincts into a genital drive is associated with the organization of an object-related orientation. The awareness of genital body ego experiences that do not require defense is represented and elaborated into fantasies of involvement with distant, unreachable new objects.

The activities of the autonomous ego functions, which have been amplified by empathic contact with an object, become increasingly complex as maturation proceeds. They are represented at the point of perceptual contact with the external world and are organized into a system of conflict-free functioning. Fantasies of expanded self-potentials are elaborated, which serve as a continuing link for enabling selective identifications. The integration of the superego is accomplished by this process of including the influence of an object within self-experience. A connection is maintained to the conflict-free sphere that creates a harmonious interrelationship with the interests of the ego and strengthens the guiding function of the superego.

The background object of primary identification establishes the foundation for all mental representation, and the firmness of its presence is reflected in the feeling of containment associated with all mental activities. The background object of primary identification is elaborated into fantasies of union with mother nature; these fantasies link to the representation of a transitional object. The containing effects of this union are evoked by contact with natural phenomena, music, beauty, and the like.

The Good Object

Good objects are the object-impression counterparts of good self-experiences and their fantasy elaborations. They are represented as an optimally gratifying object, an optimally frustrating object, and a transitional object.

The influence of a good instinctual object is represented as providing empathic, phase-specific need gratification. Orally, it is the impression of an optimally gratifying nurturer, elaborated into fantasies of an all-giving mother. With advancement into the anal phase, it is represented as an object offering optimal opportunities for exerting mastery, control, and the expression of autonomy. The fantasy of an omnipotent object establishes the linkage at the foundation of the grandiose self. Instinctual expansion into the phase of phallic exhibitionism is associated with the impression of an object's reflecting acceptance and support. Fantasies of an admiring audience are elaborated. A good genital instinctual object is represented as acknowledging genital sexuality and elaborated into fantasies of encouraging the preparation for a new object.

Optimal frustration is the impression of an object's providing optimal restraint and containment for instinctual activity. The restraint is phase-specific and is associated with empathic responses that amplify autonomous functions. The fantasy elaborations are of mirroring, which portrays an object's evoking functions in perfect attunement with self-potentials. This aspect of an object's influence reflects characteristics associated with gender, provides an effective regulatory force, and is most often selected in the process of identification. It predominates in the composition of a healthy ego ideal.

The impression of a transitional object is the nidus around which the varied impressions of a good object's influence have coalesced to form a unified entity. It is elaborated into a fantasy of transitional space, which is the psychological space that contains the mental contents of the preconscious system. This aspect of an object's influence is an integral part of the background of stability and containment that enable developmental progression and is the basic foundation upon which the superego is organized.

The Bad Self

Bad selves are the representations of instinctual overstimulation, of reactions to impingement, of sensory deprivation, and include their fantasy elaborations. Self-experiences that require defense or that are a manifestation of defense are incorporated within the entity of a bad self.

Instinctual experience that has not required defense is represented within the good self, and a line of continuity is manifested as the intensity mounts and defensive responses are instituted. That dimension of instinctual activity that is overstimulating necessitates defense and is represented within the bad self. The expansion of the component instincts and their consolidation into a genital drive have an overstimulating aspect in each phase. Orally, it is the body ego experience of greed, which is elaborated into fantasies of oral incorporation. With the emergence of anality, the body ego experience of poorly fused libidinal and aggressive drives is represented and elaborated into anal-sadistic fantasies. Phallic overstimulation is represented and elaborated into voyeuristic fantasies, as the fixation point on the introjective arm of perception is forming. The resulting stability facilitates a genital consolidation and initiates the oedipal situation. Genital overstimulation is associated with masturbatory activities and elaborated into incestuous fantasies. These fantasies are accompanied by defensive responses that facilitate their structural linkage to the impression of an overstimulating object. A new object-related boundary for the unconscious system is formed, in conjunction with the structured linkage of primal scene fantasies to the representation of genital overstimulation. The conflict engendered by these genital fantasies has an organizing influence that fosters the integration of the superego into an effective regulatory agency.

Reactions to impingements are nondiscriminatory and involve withdrawal from the source of impingement. During the narcissistic phases of development, they had been utilized to establish a boundary for unconscious mental activity. In a genital organization, they are available for defensive responses, and their fantasy elaborations of fight, flight, and withdrawal establish unions that are responsive to the superego regulation of repression proper.

The body ego experiences of sensory deprivation are represented as unrealized self-potentials. They are elaborated into a fantasy of emptiness that is particularly effective as a defensive response to instinctual overstimulation.

The Bad Object

Bad objects are the object-impression counterparts of bad self-experience and their fantasy elaborations. They are the influences of an object that elicit a defensive response and are represented as an instinctually overstimulating object, an impinging object, and a depriving object.

The representation of an overstimulating instinctual object is the portal of entry of instinctual demand. It reflects the traumatic dimension on the continuum of biophysiologic demand, has an intensity with the independent qualities of an object, and is in need of the greatest degree of defensive regulation. This instinctual aspect of the bad object is represented in accord with the phase of instinctual expansion that is in the ascendency. During each pregenital phase, it is represented as a source of danger that must be avoided. Consequently, the flow of instinctual activity toward representation within self-experience is constantly interrupted by the potential vulnerability to trauma. This is reflected in the fantasy elaborations, which are variations on the theme of a primal scene. The primal scene is a hidden, ominous, mysterious instinctual presence (the self with object qualities), which is overstimulating to the point of trauma. Primal scene fantasies may be shaped or affected by interactions with the external world, but these experiences are not a necesary condition for their development. When a genital consolidation is attained, cohesiveness, continuity of experience, and object constancy are sufficiently advanced that the influences of an object can be organized to regulate the impact of the self with object qualities. The impression of an overstimulating genital instinctual object is elaborated into a primal scene fantasy that is structurally linked to self-experiences of genital overstimulation. For the first time, a pathway is formed that insures a continuous influx of instinctual demand. The oedipal conflict has formed two new structures to link the systems of representation at the interior that bear a resemblance to each other. One links the impression of a bad instinctual object through its primal scene fantasy to the experiences of instinctual overstimulation and forms a structured pathway of integration. The other links the representation of instinctual overstimulation through its incestuous fantasy to the impression of a bad instinctual object and forms a new boundary for the unconscious system. This distinction is significant because the expression of primal scene fantasies reflects a movement toward instinctual integration, and the expression of incestuous fantasies is indicative of defensive activity.

The impinging impressions of a bad object are affected by the impact of instinctual impingements, which are reflected in their fantasy elaborations. The fantasies are of destructive threats in accord with the stage of psychosexual development in which they have formed—orally as cannibalistic, anally as sadistic, phallically as humiliating, and genitally as castrating. The fixation point, on the projective arm of perception, is originally based on a recognition of the good object's bad qualities during the anal period. This was a perception of the line of continuity of prohibitive experience, extending from the optimally frustrating impressions of a good object through prohibitions to the impinging impressions of a bad object. The fixation point expands and is depersonified, which changes the nature of its attachment to an object. The continuity of prohibitive experience is also the perceptual pathway for identifications with an aggressor when the prohibitive influence of an impinging object must be included within self-experience. Identifications with an aggressor create reaction formations in the self-system and establish prohibitive superego functions at that locale.

The impressions of nonempathic, sensorily depriving qualities in an interaction are represented as a depriving object. They are elaborated into fantasies of an object possessing those attributes that are deficient as a result of the deprivation. Depending upon the internal conditions, the fantasies portray the object as provocatively withholding or as idealized.

Superego Regulation of the Pathway of Instinctual Integration

The perceptual recognition of an external object's having independent objects of its own is a manifestation of sufficient structuralization to represent the influx of biophysiologic demand and include its unseen dimensions. The establishment of this structural pathway for the integration of instinctual demands has enabled a shift in perspective, from a narcissistic to an object-related orientation. A foundation is present for enlarging the capacity to represent instinctual activity and for self-expansion to continue through the effects of object-related experiences. The regulatory influence of a consolidating superego has been a crucial element in attaining this new level of psychic organization, and the superego occupies an increasingly predominant role in its ongoing evolution. The narcissistically determined structures of early developmental periods then occupy a place in the id of the dynamic unconscious, maintaining a connection to superego regulation in this realm of mental activity. These representations of narcissistic experiences add depth and individual meaning to new stimuli and serve as a reservoir for regressive, defensive responses at moments of adaptive stress. The superego exerts its restraining and prohibitive functions in regulating the influx of instinctual demand and its guiding functions in monitoring the processes of selective identification, sublimation, depersonification, and the activities of the conflict-free sphere of the ego.

The pathway of instinctual integration is initiated by passage through the id of the dynamic unconscious. At its most advanced genital level of organization, it is represented as an instinctually overstimulating object and is elaborated into primal scene fantasies. During the oedipal period, these primal scene fantasies have been structurally linked to the representations of genital overstimulation. An uninterrupted pathway for the representation of instinctual demand within the self-system has thereby been established. The final step on this pathway of integration is negotiated, when the self-experiences of genital overstimulation no longer require defense and can be included within good self-experience.

The oedipal conflict instigates an acceleration in selective identifications, which are increasingly discriminating and strengthen the functional capacities of good self-experience. Instinctual activity, which had been overstimulating and represented within bad self-experience, is now capable of representation without the need for defense. Secondary autonomy has been attained, and these good instinctual self-experiences are available for sublimatory activities and to serve as a boundary for the conflict-free sphere.

Primal scene fantasies, reflecting unconscious instinctual activities, are expressed through the formation of their derivatives in the preconscious system. The grandiose self, forming the inner perceptual border of the superego, monitors the effects of primary-process activity and registers the mental contents evoked in the preconscious system. Defensive responses, formed by unions of sensory deprivation and reactions to impingement with their object-impression counterparts, are activated by the signaling and regulatory functions of castration anxiety. They are especially effective in modulating the effects of overstimulation, by engaging perceptual attention and reinforcing repression proper. The ego ideal, forming the outer perceptual border of the superego, monitors the effects of secondary-process activity and registers the mental contents evoked in the transition from the preconscious to conscious systems.

In the early phases of superego organization, its functions are polarized. A prohibitive function is exercised at one pole where the system of self-experiences has been represented and an idealizing function at another pole where the system of object impressions has been represented. Selective identifications strengthen the self-system, abet the integration of instinctual activity, and diminish the need for compensatory idealizations and excessive prohibition. The multiple functions of the superego are consolidated and operate in harmony with the conflict-free sphere, which is organizing into a system of functions at the periphery. Concurrently, the alterations in the fixation points that are taking place facilitate discrimination in selecting the influences of an object that are included within self-experience. The process of depersonification on the projective arm of perception expands the range of attachments to an object that maintains differentiation and loosens the tie to narcissistic influences. The integration of the fixation point on the introjective arm of perception enables new object-related experiences to be self-enhancing. The superego assumes a more dominant role in guiding the choice of sublimatory activities and external interactions. Primitive, archaic, and narcissistic structures take their place deeper in the personality, where they give emphasis to the individual's uniqueness, strengthen cohesiveness, and more firmly ground the sense of personal identity.

The healing of splits in the superego results in the functions of prohibition, idealization, regulation, and guidance operating in concert with each other and with the ongoing activities of the ego. Repression proper is more effective, and instinctual demand can be defended at its source. Kohut (1971) offered a definition of the healthy narcissism of the "bipolar self." He described it as the establishment of ambitions and goals at the pole of mirroring, guided by the morals and standards at the pole of idealization, in the utilization of the individual's talents and skills. This definition can also apply to a healthy functioning superego, operating as an independent agency, in harmony with the capacities and interests of the ego.

The formation of fixation points on the projective and introjective arms of perception, of the grandiose self and ego ideal into perceptual structures that provide boundaries within which the superego can organize, and of the structure of castration anxiety all have been necessary for the oedipal conflict to flourish and function as a psychic organizer. The elaboration of oedipal fantasies has formed new structures insuring cohesiveness at the interior and enabling object relatedness. The oedipal conflict is resolved through selective identifications, as the superego assumes the functions of regulation, restraint, and guidance. The processes of depersonification on the projective arm of perception, of integration of the fixation point on the introjective arm of perception, and of defining the boundaries of a conflict-free sphere proceed more rapidly. The ebb and flow and continued evolution of these interrelated psychological processes occupy the developmental period of latency.

Discussion

A's anally influenced genitally determined instinctual demands gradually became more integrated, and the anxiety signaling a need for defense abated. The harsh, punitive, prohibitive influences of an object, which provided regulation, were also diminished. He displayed an increasing capacity to represent and sublimate instinctual activity, was able to recognize good and bad qualities in both the self and object, and self-regulatory functions were available that could be sustained with a level of freedom from the influence of external objects. He was able to think of himself as the driver of his own car, could recognize the weaknesses and limitations of his regulatory functions, and could imagine a way to negotiate the adaptational demands of his inner and outer worlds.

Accompanying this emerging function of self-regulation was a budding ability to be selective in the kinds of interactions that fostered continued developmental progression. This was manifested in his choice of activities. He chose football as a vehicle for the more sublimated expression of his aggressive drives. A perceived football as an opportunity to discharge aggression in a safe and contained manner. He then chose track as an activity that was more consonant with his particular skills and abilities. As he stated, he could be both part of a group and separate from it, and his determination could compensate for the deficiencies in his level of skill. A could now perceive a relationship between interactions with external objects and his inner capacities and select those that were enhancing. The regulatory and guiding functions of his evolving superego were operating in concert with each other, and with his ego interests.

A was also showing evidence of directing perceptual attention to the source of a stimulus. Earlier, when confronted with instinctual activity exerting a demand for perceptual attention in the self-system, he found it necessary to direct attention to the representations of a depriving or impinging object. Now, he was recognizing the emergence of instinctual overstimulation and could institute a defensive response.

Selective identifications were noticeable, as he included the influences of an object he admired within self-experience. A identified with football players capable of violence in a contained and sublimated fashion. This was associated with a transformation of his wishful self-imagery into more realistic self-imagery. He fantasied himself as a super football player with agility and compared this image with his limitations, awkwardness, and deficiencies. It was not experienced as a narcissistic injury but as a further step that aided him in an adequate selection of activities that would enhance his growth. Selective identifications played a significant role in the resolution of *A*'s oedipal conflict. They amplified his feeling of masculinity and made him feel strong enough to engage in heterosexual relationships. He could perceive the female as a potential object choice, rather than a source of injury and damage.

The shift from narcissism to object relatedness had previously been noted. This shift was even more apparent in *A*'s search for relationships, in which he could feel a part of the group, rather than feeling isolated from the group. The feeling of belonging was a reflection of this newly formed capacity. He could now feel enhanced by virtue of enagement with an external object. Previously, the meaning of a relationship was determined solely by the effect it had upon him. This aspect was also apparent in the therapeutic interaction. Therapy was important to *A* in new and different ways. It was no longer a matter of life and death when the therapist was momentarily blind to the meaning of his unconscious communciations. He showed a growing ability to represent his experiences in a fuller and more elaborate fashion. He could provide derivative expressions of unconscious perceptions that were easier to understand and guided the therapist more effectively. There was more leeway for *A* to absorb the narcissistic injury associated with the discovery of inner truths and the narcissistic injuries associated with the therapist's periodic lapses in empathy. *A* was able to indicate the value of the relationship and did not have to deny or avoid the emergence of aggression toward the therapist.

The early superego precursors had been fragmented, destructive, and experienced as frightening, prohibitive images. They had now been modulated by the influence of the therapeutic interaction and organized into an internal agency providing regulation, restraint, and guidance. In the initial contacts, *A*'s internal dialogue was carried on with split-off aspects of self-experience and of an object's influence. These were perceived as separate entities. Now, internal dialogue was present in the form of thought and language. This was manifested by his approach to inner exploration. *A* entered each session and examined the contents of his conscious system. This act of self-observation was based on the functioning of the eye of consciousness. Periodically, he would note an inner reaction that gradually emerged as an underlying fantasy. The fantasy appeared to be registered by an inner perceptual focus, which was consonant with the concept of a superego eye. This shift in perceptual focus, from the activity of the superego eye to the activity of the eye of consciousness, was also evident in the process of transforming wishful self-imagery into realistic self-imagery.

J exhibited a very harsh, punitive, and sadistic superego response to any instinctual activity. This was demonstrated in the extreme quilt he experienced in revealing his excitement at the funeral of his grandparents. The sadistic instinctual meaning of his excitement had mobilized the restraining, prohibitive force of an internally represented aggressor. However, this prohibitive superego function was largely ineffective, which required the formation of symptomatic compromises in an effort to achieve regulation. Though his superego was functional, it was harsh, inadequately organized, and continued to require reinforcement from external objects.

The intensity of anally influenced genital oedipal conflicts had prevented any significant degree of resolution. Consequently, the developing superego remained fixated in its early stages. Feelings of inadequacy, shame, and guilt were a constant inner presence, reflected J's identifications with a sadistic aggressor, and were mobilized in response to poorly controlled sadistic aggression.

J attempted to utilized his thinking process to master instinctual activities. Aggressive and poorly fused libidinal drives were expressed in the compromises of his symptoms; that is, a fear of the destruction of his family and the sexual overtones in his fear of reading (the next word he read might be overstimulating). Anally determined reaction formations dominated his adaptation to all stimuli. He was neat, orderly, and conforming in his behavior and worked very hard to not be seen as aggressive. Although J introjected new experiences, indicating that the introjective arm of perception was open, it was the result of a regressive breakdown. New experiences were sources of overstimulation and were associated with, and regulated by, the formation of symptoms.

J's inability to resolve an oedipal conflict was consonant with the lack of integration of the varied functions of his superego. Oedipal fantasies revealed the defensive elaboration of a negative oedipal constellation. This was manifested in his homosexual play and in his sensitivity to the therapist's excitement. *J* could not tolerate the perception of his instinctual experiences. The status of the fixation point on the introjective arm of perception was expressed metaphorically in the description of his reading block. He could not tolerate the stimulus of reading and the chain of associations that it evoked. However, he could be read to. That is, the introjective arm of perception was open, and he could take in an interpretive statement. He feared the regressive response to a stimulus most of all.

The interpretation of *J*'s fear that the therapist was aroused by his inner revelations and unable to contain the excitement evoked an image in *J* of a sexually provocative mother and an enraged father. *J* felt contained by the interpretation and could allow himself to perceive a woman as a genital sexual object. An immediate prohibitive response was elicited, which was indicative of the extreme conflict engendered by his oedipal situation. Object-related experiences were a threat, rather than being enhancing. Superego functions were dominated by a need for harsh restraint and were not integrated to operate in harmony with *J*'s ego interests. Any instinctual expression was accompanied by the anticipation of a sadistic attack.

The various symptoms of compulsive counting, intrusive ideation, rituals, and hand-washing compulsions were all manifestations of an intensely conflicted internal dialogue. The mental contents perceived by the eye of consciousness were in constant opposition to those perceived by the superego eye.

CHAPTER 9

Significance of the Latency Period

Introduction

The period of latency usually has reference to a chronological segment of time from the ages of 5 or 6, to the ages of 11 or 12. The term *latency* has been applied to this time period because there appeared to be an abatement of open evidence of instinctual intensity. At one time, there was even a question as to whether there was a physiological component to the supposed diminution of drive activity. The active instinctual involvements of early childhood appeared to change in their intensity and manner of expression during this time, until the upsurgence of instinctual activity with the onset of pubescence. Many observers have questioned the idea of an abatement of sexual activity, and there is ample evidence to support this view. Sublimated expressions of instinctual activity are abundantly present in children whose development has been unimpeded by arrests, deficiencies, or pathological distortions, which are associated with an internal capacity for more effective regulation.

The psychological functioning characteristic of latency includes an increase in sublimatory activities, a flourishing of fantasy and symbolic productions, an increase in the identifications with parents and significant others, and the emergence of moral standards and values. In addition, the defensive organization of the ego is more in evidence, more effective and consistent, with a predominant focus upon the use of repression proper.

Latency can also be defined in relation to the status of the oedipal situation, the level of superego organization, and the degree of independence from the regulatory influence of external objects. The onset of latency is then equated with the onset of resolution of the oedipal conflict, and a fuller resolution, along with a consolidation of the superego into an independent agency, is the intrapsychic task of this developmental phase. When defined by these criteria, there are a considerable number of children who do not experience a period of latency. Pathological influences have interfered with their development and prevented the elaboration of an oedipal conflict or interfered with its resolution. There are also children whose development has been arrested or delayed or who have manifested these characteristics at a much later chronological age. *A*, for example, was such a child. The period of latency emerged well after the physiological changes and capacity for genital discharge of pubescence had been in evidence. This would indicate that the characteristics of latency are an expression of the psychological changes associated with the formation and resolution of an oedipal conflict. The oedipal situation reflects the shift from narcissism to object relatedness, and the emergence of a consolidated, independently functioning superego is intimately interrelated with the degree of oedipal conflict resolution.

In this chapter, I will focus attention on the developmental processes that occupy the latency period. It is a time when the new structures that have formed from the organizing function of the oedipal conflict are stabilized, the varied superego functions are integrated into an independent agency, and the points of fixation are altered for new object-related experiences to enhance self-expansion.

Clinical Material

A continued to engage in the process of inner exploration. He entered each session and directed his attention to the thoughts and feelings that occupied his mind. The following session is illustrative. He began by talking about his parents and brother, in depth. He described various events and enlarged upon their meaning. He perceived his father's anger as an expression of helplessness and frustration. *A* now experienced moments of warmth and responsiveness with his father and recognized the pain his father had suffered in his life. He was helpful in teaching *A* to drive, yet short tempered when *A* made a mistake. He portrayed his mother's efforts to respond to him with warmth and spoke of his irritation in response to her whining attitude. Often this elicited an appeasing response in *A* and made him feel controlled and submissive. He also saw his mother as someone to turn to for help, when he was confused. This was in contrast to his father who quickly lost his patience. He depicted playful moments with his brother, who he both envied and admired. *A*'s brother began to emerge as a person who had significance. Previously, he was seen only as an annoying presence. *A* and his brother were together in opposition to parental restraints, which gave him a feeling of involvement and sharing. Interspersed with these descriptions were many allegories that expressed a new awareness of the varied qualities in his relationships. *A* then recalled episodes with the therapist, in which there had been differing experiences. In some, *A* had been understood, in some the therapist had been confused, and in some there had been an empathic lapse. He utilized analogies that vividly portrayed their meaning. The therapist participated by validating *A*'s recollections and adding his own inner reactions. *A* then thought of stories concerning people who had reached a point in their lives when they were making a decision to go off on their own. The therapist commented that *A* seemed to be putting his life in perspective and thinking about a time when he would be leaving his therapy. *A*'s response was to recall the times when the experience of being away from therapy filled him with panic. He then remembered the dream when he had been constructing a new building and was looking for the top floor. He felt a time was coming when he would complete his therapy, for in his recall of the dream, he imagined a top to the building.

K was a 6-year-old girl, referred due to her parents' concern about her extreme tension and unhappiness and her school's concern about her performance. She appeared to have very high potentials and was doing poorly. She was described as bright, driven and perfectionistic. She had recently developed an eye tic that had triggered the referral. *K* was overstriving, underachieving, and there was a constant feeling of tension in her presence.

The slightest frustration would eventuate in an angry outburst or in *K*'s berating herself and stating that she wanted to die. *K* resisted coming to her first appointment but reluctantly complied with her parents' insistence.

She appeared overly prim and proper, sat immobile, and periodically displayed an eye-blinking tic. She spoke in an overly mature fashion about herself, her relationships with those close to her, and of her involvement with school and various activities. She worked hard to present a picture of herself as a competent, adequate little girl who was perfectly content with her life. The therapist's impression was of a tightly wound spring, and he expressed this to *K*. She responded by giggling and stated, ''That's silly, people can't be like springs.'' *K* thought the therapist was weird. *K*'s reaction made the therapist feel that he had established an empathic connnection to some inner longing that had to be kept tightly in check. At the end of the session, the therapist stated that he thought *K* had shown him a picture of her outsides and that it might be important to meet regularly to know what was inside. *K* responded again by giggling and stating that that, too, was silly. All that people had inside was a heart and lungs. As *K* spoke, her whole manner relaxed, she became more spontaneous in her movements and readily agreed to meet on a regular basis.

In the early hours, she was eager to come and enthusiastic in her approach to the therapist. She became increasingly spontaneous in her behavior and verbal expressions. She appeared to be full of vitality. Her overly mature manner gradually dissolved, and she revealed a wide range of emotional reactions. These initially centered around her descriptions of school, extracurricular activities, and interactions with peers. She spoke of children and situations she hated, loved, envied, and admired. She hated school and especially the effort and concentration that was demanded. She longed to sit by the TV, watch cartoons, and be free of any demand for production. She saw her teachers as the source of these demands and visualized them silently looking at her in intensely disapproving ways. This immediately triggered thoughts of children being wild and out of control, which led them into situations of danger. The therapist thought of *K*'s fear of her instinctual drives and of the prohibitive inner responses that were designed to effect control. These inner prohibitions were simultaneously enormously inhibiting.

Periodically, a hunger to be nurtured and comforted would surface, as K sought relief from the conflicts she experienced. This was poignantly expressed as K was describing her inability to fall asleep. She felt restless and frustrated, like having an itch that she needed to scratch but being unable to reach it. She was reminded of the movie, *Lord of the Flies*. It was scary to think of a situation where all structure and rules were absent. The therapist related K's concern to her experience in therapy. The aura of encouragement made her feel overstimulated, which mobilized prohibitions that were very strict and disapproving. She seemed to be asking the therapist to provide rules and structure that could offer protection. K immediately responded by talking about her wish to be just like her father. He always seemed to handle everything and had an answer to any problem. The following session occurred shortly afterward.

K began by talking about how much she knew and how capable she was. She had brought an advanced book to demonstrate to the therapist how well she could read. She then wrote several complicated words to show how well she could spell. As she did so, it was evident that she misread and misspelled various words. K's attitude was one of emphasizing how right she was and challenging the therapist to point out her mistakes. The therapist stated that K seemed to be questioning whether the therapist would tell her things that he could see were wrong and help her face inner uncertainties. K first became angry and proclaimed that she was right and she knew it. She then put the book down to show the therapist gymnastic tricks that she had learned. She emphasized how much more adept she was then her sister, though her sister was several years older. K became embarrassed and softly referred to the envy and admiration she felt for her sister. She hesitantly admitted that she was always striving to beat her sister and was unable to do so. She felt driven to show everyone that she could do everything well, and when she could not, she felt intensely frustrated and began to hate herself. K's attitude toward the therapist shifted, and she teasingly asked if he could do the gymnastic feats she was doing. She proceeded to demonstrate, commenting on how impossible these tasks were for the therapist to accomplish. K thought the therapist was too clumsy and awkward, felt disappointment that he could not do these things, and wished he was more agile. The therapist reflected on his having missed the significance of K's communication; she had wanted the therapist to see how she did not feel complete without a penis and was disappointed when the therapist could not help her see that.

K became pensive and suddenly remembered a dream. She was in her bedroom with her mother and father. A monster threatened to break into the room. She felt she had to protect her mother, who was awkward and clumsy. Her father disappeared, but she knew he was okay. The dream made her think of her mother and how much she missed her after school. She then fantasied being in her mother's lap watching TV and softly spoke of her disappointment in her mother. There was a contemptuous tone in her voice as she described her mother's ineptness. The therapist stated that he was reminded of K's feeling about the therapist's ineptness, and how this feeling barely covered a deeper feeling about the therapist that seemed like the monster in the dream. K became secretive, as she was flooded with thoughts that were embarrassing. She did not know if she could say them. She gradually revealed her fantasies about sexual activities, which were interspersed with comments on how bad her words were. She excitedly recalled giggling with her girlfriends about using bad words. She went on to elaborate upon her wish to have a boyfriend, and of her interest in various boys. She stopped, felt embarrased, and alluded to her curiosity about male genitals.

The Developmental Tasks of Latency

The period of latency is introduced as identifications are specifically selected to achieve a resolution of the oedipal conflict. The superego is gradually established as the primary regulatory agency within the personality, and its multiple functions are integrated in harmony with the interests of the ego. Alterations in the fixation points create a degree of freedom from the influence of narcissistic attachments and enable new object-related experiences to be represented. The superego assumes dominance in guiding the choice of interactions that will foster increasingly discriminating selective identifications. It is through the agency of an integrated superego that the individual utilizes talents and skills, is motivated by ambitions and goals, and is guided by morals and standards. The psychic organization is preparing for the intensification of instinctual activity and the readiness for genital discharge that occur with the onset of pubescence.

The formation of the first fixation point on the projective arm of perception to maintain differentiation, of the gradiose self and ego ideal to ensure cohesiveness at the periphery, of the fixation point on the introjective arm of perception to enforce stability, and of castration anxiety for regulation are the necessary preconditions for the genital fantasies of the oedipal conflict to flourish. These genital fantasies, of instinctual overstimulation and of the instinctually overstimulating impression of an object, provide the linkages that are structuralized to insure cohesiveness at the interior. They form a new boundary for the unconscious system and a structured pathway for instinctual integration.

Instinctual demands, in traversing this pathway, ultimately attain secondary autonomy and access to sublimatory expression. The new structures that are formed to make this pathway functional establish the capacity for object-related perceptions. The unseen aspects of a stimulus must be capable of evoking body ego experiences, in order to maintain an open avenue for the influx of instinctual activity that emanates from the continuum of biophysiological demand (the self with object qualities). The response evoked by the recognition of an external object, having involvement with other unseen objects, are a manifestation of this expanded perceptual function. This reflects the shift from a narcissistic to an object-related orientation. Within a narcissistic organization, it was not possible to perceive the entire spectrum of the influx of instinctual demands.

The major thrust of latency is in the continuing resolution of the oedipal conflict, the further consolidation and integration of the superego, and in effecting alterations in the fixation points. The more advanced level of psychic organization has enlarged the capacity for instinctual representation, which is reflected in the flourishing of fantasy, the proliferation of instinctual derivatives and an increase in sublimatory activities.

The Significance of the Points of Fixation

A continuity of experience is a representational pathway in which one quality of experience gradually shades into another. The functional systems of representation have been organized into well-defined entities, in accordance with their propensity for requiring or eliciting a defensive response. With each system, good qualities of experience, or of an object's influence, are separated from bad qualities. The separation is not complete, as lines of continuity of good qualities shading into bad qualities are present in both systems. In the self-system, it is a line of continuity of instinctual experience. In the object system, it is a line of continuity of prohibitive experience. The perception of these representational pathways, connecting good and bad qualities, has a stabilizing effect that enables the formation of structural unions between the self- and object systems. This recognition of good and bad qualities forms a fixation point, which then exerts an influence upon the further perception of stimuli. When the fixation point results from recognizing the line of continuity of prohibitive experience, it is based upon an infantile attachment to an object and forms on the projective arm of perception. When it results from recognizing the line of continuity of instinctual experience it is based upon the infantile experiences at the time of recognition and forms on the introjective arm of perception. Although the fixation points provide the necessary stability for new structures to form, they limit the range of new experiences by creating a fixed manner of perceiving all stimuli. Thus, when the new structures are solidified, it is essential for the fixation points to undergo changes that can support the influx of new experiences and maintain their differentiating function.

The fixation point on the projective arm of perception, based on the good object's bad qualities, anchors object constancy and differentiation. The stabilizing influence enables unifying and differentiating structures to develop. The grandiose self is formed to balance the experience of vulnerability associated with separateness, and the ego ideal is formed to include influences of an object within self-experience. The grandiose self and ego ideal form perceptual boundaries within which the superego can organize and a focused area of perceptual activity that is on a continuum with the eye of consciousness (the superego eye).

The process of selective identification, involved in structuring the ego ideal, directs perceptual attention into the self-system during the phallic phase of psychosexual development. A fixation point is then formed on the introjective arm of perception, based on a recognition of the good self's bad qualities. The stability fosters the union of the lines of continuity of prohibitive and instinctual experiences that make up the structure of castration anxiety, as the component instincts consolidate into a genital drive. The conditions are present for the emerging oedipal fantasies to structuralize the foundation for a new object-related level of psychic organization, without the potentially disruptive effect of an influx of new stimuli. The fixed manner of perceiving stimuli is transiently sustained during the period of new structure formation, until the resolution of the oedipal conflict provides the wherewithal to effect changes in the fixation points.

The Significance of the Organizing Function of the Oedipal Conflict

The consolidation of the component instincts into a genital drive initiates the oedipal situation. The oedipal conflict refers to the genital fantasies that are elaborated from the representations of instinctual overstimulation and from the representation of an instinctual overstimulating object. These fantasies, of bad instinctual self-experience and of a bad instinctual object's influence, are organizing new structures at the interior that ensure cohesiveness, strengthen continuity of experience, and establish the foundation for object-related perceptions. The structuralization of bad instinctual qualities, in the self and object, makes it possible for other bad qualities to form defensive unions that aid in the regulation of overstimulation. The conflict engendered motivates and accelerates the processes of selective identification that furthers the organization of the superego into an autonomous, independent regulatory agency.

Genital overstimulation is represented as a facet of bad self-experience and is elaborated into incestuous fantasies. The portal of entry of instinctual demand is represented as a provocative, seductive, genital sexual object. The incestuous fantasies are linked to this object impression to form a structure that functions as the boundary of the id of the dynamic unconscious. The primal scene fantasies, which are elaborated from this impression of a bad instinctual object, are linked to the representations of genital overstimulation. This linkage forms a firm structural connection from the portal of entry of instinctual demand in the object system, to instinctual experiences requiring defense in the self-system. An uninterrupted pathway is established for the continuous flow of instinctual demand into the realm of self-experience. Previously, it was readily disrupted, and it now can include the dimension that was unseen and unrepresentable. Instinctual activity, which is represented as an aspect of self-experience with the aid of defense, can ultimately become integrated and attain secondary autonomy. For this step to be negotiated, the representations of good self-experience must be strengthened. Instinctual demands that were overstimulating, required defense, and were represented as a facet of bad self-experience can then be represented within the good self.

The increase in instinctual intensity accompanying a genital consolidation creates a potential for advances in the degree of integration and for the amount of overstimulation that is present. The organizing influence of the oedipal conflict is manifested throughout the personality, in forming new structures to support object relatedness, in providing the impetus for organizing integrative forces under the aegis of a functional superego, and in motivating the formation of more effective defensive, regulatory structures. The structural union of the bad instinctual aspects of the self and object enables the other qualities of bad self-experience and of a bad object's influence to be united in the service of defense. The impression of a depriving object, elaborated into a fantasy of withholding and united with the self-experience of sensory deprivation, can attract perceptual attention to diminish the effects of overstimulation. The self-experiences of sensory deprivations are elaborated into fantasies of emptiness, which, when united with the impression of a depriving object, also aid in the regulation of instinctual overstimulation. The resolution of the oedipal conflict has strengthened good self-experience and facilitated the inclusion of greater amounts of instinctual demand. This is abetted by the ascendency of the superego as an effective, regulatory agency, which enhances the incentive and capacity for successful, discriminating selective identifications.

The Significance of the Healing of Superego Splits

Within a genitally determined psychic organization, cohesiveness and object constancy are secured, and there are well-established lines of continuity of experience. A given stimulus, emanating from the internal world or originating in the external world, resonates and is registered throughout the personality. Perceptual boundaries exist that define the varied systems of consciousness. Conscious, preconscious, and unconscious mental activities operate under different regulatory principles, creating differences in the way that a stimulus is experienced. Each realm of consciousness has a differing structural composition with differing degrees of neutralized energy available and reactive resonance with focused areas of perceptual activity that monitor, regulate, and determine the meaning of a stimulus.

A split in the superego refers to a polarization of its functions and is manifested by the activity of repression proper. In the initial stages of superego organization, repression proper functions by directing perceptual attention away from what is most threatening and toward that which is least threatening. However, each has continuity with the other. The influx of instinctual intensity, accompanying the elaboration of an oedipal conflict, evokes a threat of overstimulation within the self-system. A need is present, at that locale, for the restraining, prohibitive influences of an object. This is accomplished by a process of identification with the aggressor and results in the superego's prohibitive function's being exerted at the pole where self-experiences are represented. The idealizing function of the superego is expressed in the fantasies that are elaborated to compensate for deficiencies in self-experience. This function is exerted at the pole where the object impressions are represented. The regulatory function of the superego is reflected in the selective identifications that strengthen self-experience and resolve the oedipal conflict. The superego monitors the selection of those identifications that are necessaary for the integration and sublimation of instinctual demands, as the need for compensatory idealizing fantasies and severe prohibition abates. The regulatory function of the superego gains dominance, repression proper is able to utilize the capacities for restraint and defense at the source of a stimulus, and the splits in the superego are healed.

Identifications occur along a pathway, structured by the ego ideal, which forms an outer boundary of the superego. It is regulated by the reality principle and perceptually attuned to secondary process mental activities. Idealizations occur along a pathway, structured by the grandiose self, which forms an inner boundary of the superego. It is regulated by the pleasure principle and is perceptually attuned to primary process mental activities. As repression proper gradually becomes more effective, the varied superego functions operate in unison and harmony with the interests of the ego. The superego continues to exert a prohibitive function to support the effectiveness of repression proper and a guiding function to monitor the discriminatory selection of necessary identifications, new experiences, and sublimatory opportunities. The focused areas of perceptual activity, which are incorporated in the boundaries of the superego, are organized into an internal agency of perception (the superego eye). The function of self-observation was previously exercised by the eye of consciousness alone. This focused area of perception originally evolved in locating the impressions of a good object and has only a limited ability to observe the representations of self-experience. The capacity for self-observation is enhanced and expanded by the added dimension of the superego eye. The healing of superego splits strengthens the functions of self-observation and self-criticism, by maintaining continuity and harmony between the eye of consciousness and the superego eye. When there has been an inadequate healing of splits in the superego, it is often reflected in a harsh and overly critical experience of self-observation.

The Significance of Alterations in the Fixation Points

The shift from a narcissistic orientation and the presence of an independently functioning superego providing inner direction and regulation have enabled self-expansion to continue through object-related experiences. For these experiences to transpire and be self-enhancing, changes have had to be effected in the fixation points.

The fixation point on the projective arm of perception has to be freed of the influence of infantile object attachments, and its stabilizing function has to be expanded to support mechanisms of projection and make use of more neutralized instinctual energies. The process of depersonification accomplishes this task, by symbolizing the original attachment and connecting it to the representations of new attachments. These are more under the aegis of the conflict-free sphere, follow the reality principle, and foster the growth of thought, language, and concept formation. A continuity with preconscious and unconscious areas of mental activity is maintained, as the original narcissistic attachment recedes to occupy a place in the id of the dynamic unconscious. Its stabilizing function is taken over by the representations of a good objects' bad qualities that are more advanced, object related, and secondary process oriented.

The newly developed capacity for object-related experiences, in conjunction with an increasing independence from the regulatory influence of external objects, has enabled empathic interactions to be represented within the conflict-free sphere. These are impressions of a good object's influence that are well differentiated and include an awareness of the object's independent qualities. They are containing in their effects and structured to form an outer boundary for the organizing system of conflict-free functioning. The fixation point on the projective arm of perception was initially formed by the recognition of a good object's influence but required the effects of its bad qualities to stabilize differentiation. The process of depersonification is set in motion, as the eye of consciousness registers a perceptual connection between the narcissistically determined influence of a good object at the fixation point and the object-related influence of a good object in the conflict-free sphere. This establishes a foundation for the development of symbols, thoughts, concepts, and ideas that reflect the attachment to a differentiated good object's influence. The fixation point on the projective arm of perception is thereby depersonified and expanded, which offers a solid background for projective mechanisms to function more efficiently.

The introjective arm of perception is the pathway for registering the impact of new stimuli. To the extent that a point of fixation remains, new experiences will be altered by its effects. This fixation point was formed by a recognition of the good self's bad instinctual qualities and functioned to provide the necessary stability for new object-related structures to form. The resolution of the oedipal conflict is associated with an integration of instinctual experiences that had previously required defense and results in a dissolution of the fixation point on the introjective arm of perception. The representations of phallic and genital instinctual experiences upon which it was based have attained secondary autonomy and are utilized to form an inner boundary for the conflict-free sphere. The introjective arm of perception is then open to register new stimuli from an object-related perspective, and the resulting experiences are self-enhancing. The stabilizing function of the fixation point is taken over by the conflict-free sphere.

The conflict-free sphere is an extension of the autonomous ego functions, represented as an aspect of good self-experience. It is organized into a system of conflict-free functioning at the point of perceptual contact with the external world. The inner boundary is composed of the representations of instinctual demand that have traversed the pathway of integration to attain secondary autonomy. The outer boundary is composed of the representations of a separate, well-differentiated, independent good object's influence. The processes of depersonification and instinctual integration, which have effected changes in the fixation points, are instrumental in solidifying a harmonious interrelationship between the organizing system of conflict-free functions and the regulatory, guiding functions of the superego. The ultimate fate of the self with object qualities at the interior and the object with self qualities at the periphery is to form the boundaries for a conflict-free system of ego functions.

Discussion

This brief clinical vignette is illustrative of the change in *A*'s manner of functioning and reflects the shift that has taken place from narcissism to object relatedness. *A* now displayed the capacity to perceive an object as independent and as having involvements with unseen others. His liberal use of allegories and analogies, which are depersonified and symbolized mental productions, indicated that psychological activities requiring an expanded use of projective mechanisms were now available to him. The nuances and complexities that he perceived in relationships reflected an increasing ability to register external stimuli relatively free from the influence of memories. This gave credence to the formulation that the introjective arm of perception was open and was consonant with his expanded capacity to integrate instinctual demands.

In previous sessions, the integrated functioning of *A*'s developing superego was highlighted. During this period of time, *A* was chronologically 16 years of age and was displaying psychological functioning characteristic of the latency period. He also showed a greater degree of confidence in his ability to function as a separate individual, capable of internal regulation. *A*'s derivative association to stories of people reaching a point in their lives where they could decide to be on their own was indicative of this development. It also expressed a beginning recognition that separation from psychotherapy was a logical extension of his continuing growth. The anxiety associated with separateness was contained in recollections of his earlier experiences of panic. *A*'s recall of the building construction dream, and fantasied addition of a top to the building, gave emphasis to the firmness of the new mental structures that had evolved.

K was chronologically entering the period of latency when therapeutic contact was initiated. Her manner of psychological functioning displayed some of the characteristics associated with that period. At the outset, *K* worked hard to portray herself as competent and adequate. The defensive significance of this effort was apparent in the rigidity with which she conducted herself and in the total focus upon conscious intellectual content and immediate perceptions. This aspect of her functioning gave an exaggerated and inflexible picture of qualities often associated with the latency period. There was little evidence of open instinctual activity, and the defensive organization of her ego was apparent in most of her responses. The relative absence of fantasy, instinctual derivatives, and sublimated expressions of instinctual activity were indicative of a highly conflicted internal state. Many qualities associated with latency were unavailable, having been interfered with by pathological developments. The organization of her superego was inordinately harsh, punitive, and restrictive.

In the course of the therapeutic interation, underlying genitally determined conflicts became more evident. *K* was gradually able to integrate instinctual activity more effectively, and the qualities that had heretofore been absent began to assert themselves. She then displayed a very active fantasy life, and derivatives of unconscious mental activity emerged. A wider range of emotional expression and an ability to represent a larger variety of interactions began to be manifested. Her ability to utilize intellectual functions became more effective, and she became adept at symbolically expressing her experiences. This seemed to reflect a degree of freedom from the influence of a narcissistic attachment to an object, and expansion of the fixation point on the projective arm of perception. The process of depersonification was quite limited initially and became increasingly active and effective as the intensity of her intrapsychic conflict was alleviated. The presence of pathology was indicated early in K's profound inner feeling of being disapproved of and in her concern about children being wild and out of control. Intense disappointment in, and rivalry with, the maternal figure alternated with contempt and envy and barely masked the underlying negative oedipal attachment. This defensive, transference attitude was addressed interpretively, and a threatening genital instinctual attachment to the male emerged. K had formed all of the components of an oedipal conflict. The intensity of her genital instinctual demands, in conjunction with the restricting, inhibiting effects of her defensive reactions, was interfering with its resolution and with a full integration of her developing superego. This in turn prevented the full unfolding of the processes that characterized the period of latency. The fixation point on the introjective arm of perception was defensively maintained. K's shifting perceptions of the therapist were a reflection of the specific qualities that made up this point of fixation. Initially, the therapist was either a phallically admiring audience or a source of voyeuristic interest and disapproval. These experiences were influenced by the phallically determined fixation point on the introjective arm of perception.

The process of instinctual integration was facilitated by the effects of the therapist's interpretive interventions, and the fixed qualities of K's perceptions were gradually relinquished. The therapist was then perceived as clumsy and awkward, reflecting the negative oedipal maternal transference; he was perceived as a genital sexual object, reflecting the positive oedipal paternal transference, and as engaged with her in understanding her internal life, reflecting the openness of the introjective arm of perception to new experiences. This new capacity to perceive the therapist in varying ways, and at differing levels of perception, was a consequence of the eye of consciousness's functioning on the line of continuity with the superego eye. It was a manifestation of K's readiness to continue the thrust of progression in development and to attain resolution of her oedipal conflict. K illustrated the effects of an inordinate degree of conflict upon the full consolidation of the superego and upon the necessary alterations in the fixation points that occupy the development period of latency. As her oedipal conflict achieved resolution, it was possible for these processes to become manifested.

The thrust of the period of latency is in the continuing resolution of the oedipal conflict, the fuller consolidation of the superego, the alterations in the fixation points, the organization of a system of conflict-free ego functions, and the further elaboration of fantasies that foster the process of instinctual integration. Pathological distortions of developmental processes have a profound effect upon the manner in which mental structures are formed, and upon the manner in which stimuli are perceived. The experience of emotions are dependent upon these underlying structures, and actions are determined by the meaning of a given stimulus.

An action may be narcissistically gratifying, but if it does not have an object-related goal, it cannot be effective. The action may be a thought, an expression of individual talent or skill, or an emotion. Actions that do not involve an object are inhibited, immobilized, or ineffective. Self-experience is enhanced by the expression of talents, skills, potentials, and functions through involvement with an object. An action that is totally narcissistically determined is dominated by fantasy and exposed to potential humiliation, shame, and the destruction of its meaning. In health, emotional expressions are rich and full of meaning.

CHAPTER 10

Pubescence

Relinquishing the Attachment to Primary Infantile Objects and Their Replacement with New Objects

Introduction

The period of pubescence is associated with turmoil, crises, wide mood swings, alterations in behavior, and rapid changes in attitude, thinking, and feeling. It is a time of multiple psychological changes, intertwined with the noticeable physiological changes that are a direct consequence of hormonal activity. The developmental events that have preceded these dramatic occurrences influence the manner in which the resulting body ego experiences are represented. It is especially important to define the specific intrapsychic and interactional events of pubescence because they appear to be related to the processes involved when change is effected in a therapeutic interaction. The developmental task of pubescence is one of replacing the representations of infantile attachments to an object and attaining freedom from their influence. A psychotherapeutic process is faced with a similar task because a significant factor in the development of pathology is the tenacity with which infantile attachments are maintained. Understanding the means by which the developmental step of replacing the infantile attachment to an object is negotiated expands the view of how a therapeutic interaction can be instrumental in facilitating structural change.

Pubescence is frequently a time of intense "crushes" and hero worship. There is an intimate relationship between these experiences and the changing attitude toward infantile objects and their representations. These episodes of crushes and hero worship are reminiscent of the transference neuroses observed in the psychoanalysis of adolescents and adults. The controversy, as to whether a transference neurosis can develop in prepubescent children, continually emerges as an unsettled question. Some argue that transference manifestations are amply demonstrable in young children but that a full transference neurosis does not occur. The reasons focus upon the significance of the developing child's continuing dependency on primary objects. Others argue that a full transference neurosis is possible in prepubescent children. The child is then capable of a more appropriate dependency upon primary objects and is freed of the distortions created by a regressive transference. That is, the child is unencumbered by the regressive effects of earlier representational influences. My experience has been that, once the structural foundation necessary for a neurosis to form is present, a full transference neurosis is possible. The question as to whether it is manifested then depends upon the manner in which the therapeutic interaction is conducted. However, the experience of a transference neurosis does tend to be different in prepubescent and postpubescent children. The different is manifested in the degree of intensity, which seems to be determined by the presence or absence of a developmental need to form representations of new objects. The prepubescent child who has negotiated separation–individuation, attained cohesiveness, and is embroiled in an oedipal conflict has a minimum need for representing new objects. The postpubescent child, maintaining a tenacious attachment to the representations of infantile objects, has an intense need to form representations of new objects. In general, the prepubescent child has less of a need to replace infantile objects and more of a need to undo the fantasy distortions that interfere with healthy developmental processes. The postpubescent child has more of a need to replace infantile objects and be free of their influence in order to continue the progressive thrust of development. The crushes and hero worship of pubescence are the expression of an attachment to a new object that is designed to replace an infantile attachment. Although they display evidence of the influence the individual is seeking freedom from, there are some noticeable differences. The differences center upon the totally narcissistic quality of infantile attachments and the preoccupation with the object's well-being in both crushes and the heroes that are worshipped.

The onset of pubescence is most often identified by the first ejaculatory experience in boys and the menarche in girls. The former is an intensely instinctual experience, and the latter is an experience more linked to processes of identification. Pubescence is a period in which earlier developmental difficulties are highlighted. Marking its onset with these differing physiological changes calls attention to the idea that instinctual experiences are more in conflict in boys and that questions of identification are more troublesome in girls. This is consonant with the boy's instinctual development allowing the primary maternal object to be retained but requiring a shift in attitude, whereas the girl must shift instinctual interest from the primary maternal object to the male.

In this chapter, I will define pubescence and describe the differences in male and female development. Emphasis will be placed upon the need for replacement of infantile objects with new objects. The specific representations of an object that requires replacement will be delineated as will the processes by which this is attained. The fate of the infantile representations of the object and the role of new object representations will be outlined.

Clinical Material

A arrived late for his appointment, appearing extremely distraught. He frantically asked if he could call his mother and went on to explain that he had just had a car accident in the parking lot. His mother would kill him; he just had to call her. Could he use the phone? The therapist commented that *A* seemed to be asking whether the therapist agreed that his anxiety had to be appeased by some action. *A* continued to appear frantic and began to talk about pulling into the parking lot. He had put his foot down to stop the car and accidentally stepped on the accelerator. He then collided with the car directly facing him. There had been a loud crash, and he immediately felt overwhelmed. Someone had jumped out of the car yelling at him, a guard had run over, and a big crowd accumulated. A felt panic and was paralyzed. He gave them his name and came to his appointment. He felt totally in despair. He would never to be able to drive again. He could picture his mother's being furious with him. He felt like he had to talk to her and get some reassurance. He kept feeling the urge to pick up the phone, as he felt waves of panic about his mother's reaction. A fell silent. He then remembered having a brief thought just as he pulled into the parking space. The front of the car facing him had looked like his mother's car. The next thing that he knew was that the collision had occurred, and he felt terrified. He began to ruminate as to what would happen now. He felt the inner presence of voices screaming at him. He could really understand what people meant when they said their whole life passed before their eyes. That was exactly what it felt like. Suddenly, in a brief moment, everything that had ever happened to him seemed to pass in front of his eyes. It began with the collision and continued. He left the accident to come to his appointment, and what remained strongest was what was deepest inside. He had a feeling that if he could hold on to his view of the outside he would not feel so panicky. The panic seemed to come from losing this view. A paused again and spoke of regaining this view as he talked. He felt himself moving back to the beginning of the experience. He could see the outside event—the collision. He could see how it affected him inside. He gradually was filled with the fear of being attacked and breaking into pieces. A now appeared visibly relieved. He liked the idea of looking at himself. He remembered his thought about the other car. It was like he was crashing into his mother. The crash threatened to destroy something vital, and he was enveloped by panic. That is why he wanted to call her. He wanted to hear her voice. It seemed that if he heard her voice he would no longer be in pieces. A was amazed that, as he now thought about what happened, it did not seem so awful. He had to call the insurance company and take care of the details of the accident. The accident was not bad; it was not being able to look at himself that was bad. A paused and said, "It's like the first thing you lose is the last thing you get."

L was a 14-year-old boy, referred because his parents and school were totally frustrated in knowing how to handle and respond to him. *L* was almost always right and fiercely determined in maintaining his position. He refused to do homework because no one could provide him with a reason that was sensible to him. In addition, he could prove to the school officials that their resoning was faulty. An authoritative stance would be adopted, and *L* would mock and laugh at this attitude. The school authorities were upset that no consquences seemed to affect *L*. No matter what was tried, *L* simply smiled or laughed. At home, he was in a constant battle with his parents. In their words, he refused to face or accept reality. He had many interests and was involved in numerous projects that required intense concentration and work. However, they all were activities that he enjoyed. He totally refused to extend himself if he was not interested. He was creative and effective in what he did but only on his own terms. When given some other task, *L* would simply refuse and remain steadfast. There were also episodes of extreme temper outbursts, particularly with his mother or younger brother. These explosive responses seemed to have a large element of control. He might throw things but never hit anyone. These episodes were triggered by some injustice directed toward him. His mother felt very guilty, as *L* was frequently accurate in his perception. His father was a pragmatic individual who was not concerned with the quality of *L*'s academic performance but was deeply concerned with his inability to live "within the system." *L* was perceived as being spoiled, lazy, undisciplined, living by the dictates of his grandiosity, and unable to adapt to the world of reality. Three previous efforts had been made to seek professional help, with *L*'s refusing to return after one or two sessions. He did not resist going; he resisted returning after a short trial.

L came willingly to his first appointment. He was curious, as he had been in the past. He talked openly of his parents and school's concern. His descriptions were exactly parallel to those presented by his parents. If *L* saw a reason for doing something, he did so gladly. No one gave him valid reasons that made sense to him. Further, when he voiced his objection, no one showed him where he was wrong. They only insisted that he do as others did or that they felt it was in his best interests. He spoke of his many and varied activities. He had many friends. He valued people and relationships highly and was deeply concerned about, and sensitive to, injustice, injury, and moral values. He had found two people in his life who gave him reasons for doing things. One was a piano teacher. L played piano by ear and was pleased by his ability to play. Everyone was upset that he refused to learn to read music. They saw his talent and were angry with his refusal to develop it. He found a piano teacher who did not try to teach him music but tried to help him develop his own skills. He gave him disciplined activities to follow and explained how it could foster his own innate potentials. He also found a Hebrew teacher who explained the importance of learning Hebrew. L disciplined himself to do that, though he previously had no intention of doing so. The teacher talked to him about language as a way of solidifying a union with his forefathers. He had also talked with L of the importance of being a separate individual with his own unique thoughts. This so impressed L that he became involved in learning a new language. L then asked what the therapist thought about all that he had said. The therapist stated that L had shown qualities within himself that were expressions of his effort to be a separate individual with the strength to stand up for what he believed and to establish his uniqueness. The therapist also heard how important it was that L and the therapist see reasons for working together. The therapist wondered if L's question was expressing a sensitivity to the therapist's feeling that there was a lot left unspoken that would give a reason. (As the therapist listened to L's desperate fight to maintain his autonomy, separateness, and individuality, he was becoming aware of his own unconscious sensitivity to the underlying vulnerabilities that were unspoken.) L immediately responded by asking, "What do you mean?" The therapist stated that he meant L seemed to be fighting very hard for his autonomy but was not very effective. The therapist sensed there were things L had not spoken of that hampered him. When L told the therapist of his piano teacher and Hebrew teacher, the therapist thought he was describing what he needed from the therapist if they were to work together. L stated, "I want you to listen. There are many things I can't talk about." He then asked if that would interfere. These were things he knew about. He also knew therapy was a place where he had to talk, but he simply would not talk about some things. He was adamant in his refusal. The therapist stated that he thought L was talking about the things he did not want to—all of the time. The therapist thought *L* was asking if the therapist would ignore what he heard or not let *L* know when he heard. Much later, *L* informed the therapist that this moment was when he decided to engage in therapy. He began to feel that he could talk.

In the early months, *L* talked about his wide-ranging interests. In describing these interests, a constant theme inadvertently slipped in of *L*'s inner sense of danger, injury, and destruction. It would "slip" out, and he would make a joke of it. For example, in describing his interest in magic, he laughingly wondered what someone would do if they were missing a finger, or he wondered how a person with no arms could use a computer. On one occasion he came in tearfully and signaled the therapist to be silent. He could not talk and wanted the therapist to forget about it. He then joked about how impossible it is to forget something when someone tells you to forget it. He then hesitantly began to reveal his profound phobia. He was terrified, when he went to bed each night, that there was something in his closet. He knew it was ridiculous and made no sense. He engaged in various rituals to distract himself. *L* was totally mortified that he was so frightened. He had much trouble going to sleep. No one knew of this. He had kept it hidden, feeling it was a sign of weakness. *L* was shocked that he was telling the therapist. Now that he had, he did not know what to do about it. It made it no better or no worse. He went on to describe his fears. He had just learned of a beloved grandfather's serious illness. He felt terrified about the idea of death. This had reminded him of his phobia. He had not wanted the therapist to talk, so he could bring it up in his own way. He did not want the therapist to elicit it from him. The following session took place shortly afterward.

The therapist had received an upsetting phone call just prior to the session. *L* came in, looked at the therapist, and asked, "Do you believe in ESP?" He went on to describe his interest in ESP, telekinesis, reincarnation, and various mystic phenomena. He elaborated upon how careful he had to be as to who he talked to about it. "People think you are crazy if you believe in these events. Unless they believe in it, too, they think of you as strange. If they believe in it, then you can share your ideas and experiences." The therapist gradually became aware that he had not processed the previous phone call very well. Its effects had lingered as L entered the room (the therapist was still involved with "the craziness" of the phone call, which L had unconsciously perceived). The therapist stated he thought L sensed some inner disturbance in the therapist and was concerned that this disturbance would be attributed to L. He became silent and thought of his piano teacher. This teacher was helpful and encouraged L to play well. He went on to speak of his interest in ESP and to the things he sensed in other people. He gave many examples of coincidences that he seemed to anticipate. He reflected on how sensitive he was and how quickly he picked up on unconscious messages. L looked at the therapist and asked, "Was there something? Will you tell me?" The therapist said he thought L was checking to see if the therapist was now ready to listen because he had not been when L first came in. L had helped the therapist recognize that. L became pensive and talked of how much he has been thinking about his fear of a monster in his closet. He suddenly became aware that what he feared was inside of him, not outside of him. He had been exquisitely sensitive to things in other people. That made him feel that everything he feared was outside of him. That was what confused him about the closet. He knew there was no one there, but the fear was exactly the same as if there was someone there, and he sensed it. It made L feel there was someone hidden. Though he could not see them, they were there. He was sensing their presence, just as he sensed things unseen in other people. He was now aware, both in his sensing things in other people and in his fear of the closet, that it was connecting with something inside of him. He now felt able to think about what he feared inside of himself. The way he could do that was to look at his own thoughts the same way that he looked at another person when he tried to sense their unconscious messages. He then stated, "There is one thing I've never told you. It looks to everyone like I'm very creative and do a lot. The truth is I never complete anything." L went on to describe his coming to the end of any task and suddenly abandoning it. He felt an inner fear and tried to make it look as though he had finished, to hide the fact that he had not. "There's something about finishing a job that scares me. When I was just saying that, a song went through my head. I'll bet that's a message from inside of me." He went on to say that he felt silly and then that he knew it was not silly. "I want to be able to let things come into my mind and think about them." *L* puzzled about the song and recalled the title was "My Life." The lines had to do with someone's life being cut off. The song was bringing him a message that to finish a task was like ending his life. He felt so terrified of his life's ending that he could not complete anything. That was the feeling of something in the closet. *L* stopped and laughed, "I just had a funny thought. Someting in the closet feels like something in my mind I've kept closed off. It's trying to come out and give me a message." *L* reveled in how good it felt to think this way. He had never been able to do that. He had only been able to be afraid, pull back, and avoid thinking; then he felt humiliated about pulling away. He had never been able to think and look at what he thought about. He felt like something was expanding that let him do that. *L* then recalled his mother's telling him something that he never understood. It never made sense until just now. His mother told him that, when he was an infant, he was extremely special to her. He began to assert himself, and she became so enraged that she could not tolerate him and beat him. She hated herself for that and went into treatment. Later, when his brother was born, she involved herself with the brother in a similar way. He had reacted to the birth and early infancy of the brother with all of the reactions she thought he had from the first period of trauma. The first instance was at less than a year. The second at age 3. The intensity of his hostility to the mother made her think it was from his period of infancy. *L* recalled his mother telling him this. What he understood was that, whenever he looked at his brother, he felt like he wanted to hit him in a particular manner. He liked his brother, and it had always puzzled him. He suddenly realized that the way he wanted to hit his brother was identical to the way his mother described hitting him.

The following session occurred many months later. *L* began talking animatedly about telling several friends that he was in therapy. He recalled an earlier time when he had been fearful that someone would find out. At that time, he would have felt humiliated. Now, he values the experience more and feels comfortable in letting others know. He offhandedly laughed as he described his discovery that some others he had told were in therapy also. He paused and spoke of his new girlfriend. He met her on a trip and fell deeply in love. She lived far away, and it was extremely painful to be so in love and to be so distant. He talked with her on the phone each week and felt an intense longing afterwards. It felt to him like being on a diet and seeing your favorite food on display. Your appetite is whetted but not fulfilled. He wished he could turn it off. It was so painful. L paused and talked of being intimately connected to his girlfriend. They are able to understand each other without words. The therapist commented that, as L talked about communicating without words, it appeared to be L's way of letting the therapist know that he was talking about the therapist without words. It reminded the therapist of L's earlier fear that he would not be able to allow himself to feel such an intense attachment. L looked embarrassed and began to talk about his awareness that when he thought of turning it off he was trying to draw back. He remembered how afraid he had been of feeling love for someone. At the time, he felt he was being strong. As he looked back, it seemed like he was being defensive and closing himself up. Now he felt open to the experience and wanted to risk it. It felt good to love someone. He had an inner feeling that it must have been that way early in his life with his mother. He recalled fearing that he would never feel love for someone. The experience was difficult, but he valued it highly. He might get hurt or rejected but that seemed relatively unimportant: feeling it meant everything.

The Landmarks of Pubescence in Boys and Girls: The First Ejaculatory Experience and the Menarche

The onset of pubescence creates a new set of internal conditions, which are introduced by the manifestations of hormonal activity. These include the secondary sexual characteristics and the emergence of genital discharge and orgastic experience. The events of pubescence highlight the particular area of greatest developmental need. The boy's pubescence is dominated by the need to resolve instinctual difficulties, and the girl's pubescence by the need to resolve difficulties with identification.

For the boy entering pubescence, secondary sexual characteristics are a source of reinforcement of masculine identifications that have continued throughout the latency period. The first ejaculatory discharge is a source of intense stimulation and is evocative to those representations of self-experience in which instinctual activity was perceived as a threat. Orgastic experience involves a traversal of the pathway of instinctual integration, from the realm of biophysiology to genital discharge, in a rapid and uncontrolled though internally regulated manner. This experience stands out as a landmark that emphasizes the threat of instinctual overstimulation and the necessity for change. It is the first experience of instinctual demand (the self with object qualities), achieving genital discharge. In individuals with severe pathology, genital discharge often occurs with greater frequency and rapidity. Such individuals do not have sufficient structuralization to provide inner regulation. The orgastic experience is then superficial, fragmented, and/or panic arousing. Thus, although secondary sexual characteristics are also a manifestation of change, they are experienced as an extension of the selective identifications that have been well established during the latency period. The first ejaculatory, orgastic experience of genital discharge initiates the psychological changes of pubescence because it activates the instinctual activities that have been the area of greatest conflictual difficulty.

During the oral phase of psychosexual development, the boy's instinctual attitude toward the primary maternal object is one of seeking pleasure and avoiding displeasure. With maturation and continuing instinctual expansion into the anal phase, the boy's attitude changes to exerting efforts at domination and control or assuming a submissive posture. Movement into the phallic period is accompanied by an exhibitionistic attitude. Up to this point, the object has had only narcissistic significance. As the component instincts consolidate into a genital drive and a genital instinctual attitude begins to evolve, a sequence of intrapsychic events necessitates a shift in that attitude. The primary love object remains the same, but the instinctual aspects must be repressed. The elaboration of an oedipal conflict is associated with an intensification of instinctual activity, as the unseen dimension of biophysiological demands is accessible to representation. Castration anxiety has been structuralized to serve an essential signaling and regulatory function, which makes the boy's genital instinctual attitude an enormous threat. Under the impact of castration anxiety, a power-

ful motive is present to resolve the conflict through selective identifications. The masculine qualities of an object's influence, which,
when included within self-experience, have a strengthening effect,
are selected. The boy's instinctual life is highly conflictual, but the
resulting masculine identifications are clear and well defined. A
negative oedipal constellation is only developed when the conflict
is inordinate or when the regulatory forces in the personality are
inadequate. The degree of defensive distortion required to displace
the primary love object and establish a feminine identification is
so extreme that it is only seen as a reflection of pathology.

The girl, entering pubescence, has been more capable of instinctual integration. Increases in instinctual intensity have been
more adequately represented and less traumatic. In pubescence,
the new avenue of genital discharge has a more integrated
representational pathway to traverse and can include the representation of the mother as a primary libidinal object. However, when
the component instincts consolidate into a genital drive, the primary libidinal object presents the girl with a terrible disappointment. The mother cannot provide her with the genital gratification
that her body ego experiences demand. The genital instinctual attitude, which evolved with the mother as the primary object, is
displaced onto a male figure. This displacement to the male as a
potential source of genital gratification has not occurred as a result of a threat or trauma but as a response to disappointment. The
initial disappointments begin to include feelings of rivalry, which
makes it difficult to engage in the feminine identifications necessary for a resolution of the oedipal conflict. The process of selective identification has been more gradual and not as clearly
defined. The development of secondary sexual characteristics emphasizes the difficulties with identifications and the need for
change. The onset of the menarche initiates the psychological
changes of pubescence because it provides the impetus to further
more effective and well-defined feminine identifications.

The girl's instinctual attitude to her primary object of pleasure
and unpleasure during the oral phase and of mastery, control, and
submission during the anal phase is identical to that of the boy.
With the onset of the phallic period, changes begin to manifest
themselves. The exhibitionistic attitude is affected by the differences in the body ego experiences of genital sensations, and genital

exploration, and the emerging feeling of disappointment. A genital consolidation heightens the disappointment in the primary maternal object, which instigates a displacement of the girl's genital instinctual attitude to the father. With this displacement of genital sexual interest to a male, a rivalrous attitude toward the mother arises. A genital instinctual attachment to the mother is less of a threat and less in need of a defensive response. The experience has been one of disappointment, rather than a threat of danger or castration, and the girl is able to represent and regulate greater quantities of genital instinctual activity. A negative oedipal constellation is a developmental step, leading to a displacement to the male as a genital instinctual object. Castration anxiety, which functions to regulate this positive oedipal conflict, mobilizes responses that are more disapproving and less threatening. The disappointment abets a continuing process of differentiation from the primary maternal object, but in conjunction with the evolving rivalrous attitude, it makes feminine identifications more difficult. There is a strong motive for the girl to displace her libidinal object, whereas the impetus for establishing feminine identifications is not as imperative.

The physiological changes, associated with pubescence, highlight earlier developmental difficulties. These center around instinctual experiences in the boy, and identifications in the girl. For this reason, the psychological changes of pubescence are initiated with the first ejaculatory episode in boys and with the menarche in girls.

The Grandiose Self and Ego Ideal in Pubescence

The events that have been occurring during latency have been important in preparation for the rapid and profound changes that occur during the period of pubescence and adolescence. The increasing autonomy of the superego, the process of depersonification on the projective arm of perception, the integration of the fixation point on the introjective arm of perception, and the formation of boundaries for a conflict-free system of ego functions have all continued during latency. There has been an increasing degree of self-differentiation and a measure of independence from the influence of narcissistically determined attachments to infantile objects. The major perceptual structures of the grandiose self and ego ideal, which form the boundaries of the superego, have continued to be maintained by the representations of these primary infantile attachments. Although the developments of the latency period have established a foundation for continuing progression in differentiation and separateness, the object attachments that comprise these major perceptual structures exert an influence in perpetuating an infantile attitude toward new experiences and new relationships. They also have an affect upon the defensive responses that are utilized and upon the ongoing process of selective identification.

The combination of a rapid influx of genital instinctual demand with emphasis on genital discharge and the rapid body changes associated with the increased hormonal activity of the pubescent period instigates a potential state of trauma. The sudden increase in intensity of instinctual demand mobilizes an urgent need for defensive responses, which are based upon infantile attachments to the restraining and prohibitive influences of an object. The activation of these narcissistically determined regulatory forces is in opposition to the progressive movement of attaining greater freedom from their influence. The latency child has attained the capacity for receiving new perceptions that are object related in nature and are self-enhancing. The continuing maturation of ego functions and ever-widening involvement with varied external objects all reflect this new perceptual relationship. The onset of pubescence places these advanced experiences of autonomy, differentiation, and individuation in jeopardy. In the male, it is initiated with the first ejaculation, and in the female with the menarche. The male has had a stronger motive for masculine identifications designed to strengthen self-experience but is less able to integrate instinctual activity. The female has established a more effective pathway of instinctual integration but is less able to strengthen self-experience through feminine identifications.

The intensification of instinctual demand and bodily changes that emerge in pubescence puts stress upon the object-related perceptions of the outer and inner worlds that have consolidated during latency. For further advancement in independence and autonomy to eventuate, it is necessary that the primary narcissistic attachments to infantile objects be relinquished and replaced. The grandiose self and ego ideal have established the perceptual boundaries of the superego and thus have access to the perceptual contact with the external world that is required for the process of replacement to take place. Were this not to occur, superego functions would continue to be affected by infantile experiences. The attachment to new independent objects exerts an influence that is more expressive of an object-related, reality-oriented perspective. The superego function of guidance and direction, interrelated with the conflict-free sphere, will then be in harmony with the interests of the ego in the ultimate selection of a love object, a work life, and activities for sublimation. The original narcissistically determined structure of the grandiose self and ego ideal can then function solely to maintain the boundary of the preconscious system of mental activity.

The Conditions for Replacement of Infantile Attachments to an Object

The primary task of the period of pubescence is in relinquishing an attachment to the representations of narcissistically determined infantile objects and replacing them with the representations of new and independent objects. The processes and structures involved in that replacement are of particular significance because this is the developmental foundation for the structural changes that occur in a psychoanalytic process. The grandiose self and ego ideal were originally formed to structurally unite the self- and object systems of representation. They have evolved to establish boundaries, within which the superego has organized into an independently functioning agency. These structures are composed of the representations of infantile narcissistic attachments to an object that reflects the advancement from narcissism to object relatedness. The grandiose self involves the attachment to a fantasied object's omnipotence and reflects the earliest experiences of separateness. The ego ideal involves the attachment to the influences of an object that strengthens self-experience and reflects the movement toward self-regulation. These infantile attachments continue to exert an influence upon the superego's multiple functions, and it is thus essential for them to be replaced.

The resolution of the oedipal conflict has resulted in the consolidation of the superego as a functional agency, independent from the influences of the external world. In order to be fully independent, the superego must also be free of the narcissistic influence of infantile attachments. This internal agency enforces repression, regulates the instinctual pathway of integration, provides guidance in the selection of those identifications that further developmental progression, and gives expression to the morals and standards that regulate the ego's adaptive interactions with the external world. The superego monitors all psychic functioning to attain a harmonious balance between narcissistic self-enhancement and object-related self-expansion.

Pubescence is the entry into the adolescent period where the final steps are taken for the development of a genital character. This refers to an advanced level of psychic organization in which all stimuli are registered without distortion and resonate throughout the personality to be given individual meaning. A genital character formulates ambitions and goals, utilizing talents and skills shaped by morals and standards, in the expression of actions. These actions (affects, thoughts, behavior) reflect the effects of sublimation, the attainment of secondary autonomy, and the flexible utilization of varying levels of neutralized energy. This occurs on a background of cohesiveness, object constancy, and a well-integrated sense of identity. It is important that the representations of narcissistically determined experience do not influence the dominance of secondary-process thinking, the choice of new love objects, or the selection of new identifications. It is equally important that these narcissistic representations remain available as an integral part of the pathway of instinctual integration and to provide depth and meaning to new experiences.

The definitive step in the organization of a genital character necessitates the replacement of the infantile attachments to an object that comprise the structures of the grandiose self and ego ideal, with the representations of new and independent objects. The representations of these new object-related attachments must maintain a connection to the process of depersonification on the projective arm of perception and to the representations of self-experience that had constituted a fixation point on the introjective arm of perception and attained secondary autonomy. The connection is created in the process of replacement, which results in a grandiose self and ego ideal that are restructured to be independent of an infantile, narcissistic influence. The primary infantile structures can then take their place in the final organization of the id of the dynamic unconscious and maintain a boundary for the preconscious system.

In pubescence, there is a developmental need for new experiences with new external objects. They provide the body ego experiences and object impressions that, when represented under the proper conditions, are utilized for replacement of the original infantile attachments to an object. For the process of replacement to be initiated, the new experiences must be reminiscent of the conditions under which the infantile attachments (that comprise the original structures) were represented. The superego guides this process and is selective of interactions that most closely parallel those conditions. This necessitates a search for, and recreation of, interactions with new external objects that meet the regressive conditions required to resonate with the structures of the grandiose self and ego ideal. In this way, the period of separation–individuation is recreated in active interactions with new external objects. It could be described as regressive in nature, but it is in the service of development. The regressive conditions of the new interaction facilitate the dominance of the infantile attachments and simultaneously expose them to be registered by the eye of consciousness. This focused area of perceptual activity is an expression of the integrative forces within the conscious system and establishes a bond with the conflict-free system of functions. The ongoing process of depersonification and instinctual integration is extended to participate in the representation of these new object-related attachments and to distinguish them from their infantile counterparts. The result is in a gradual relinquishing of the narcissistic attachment, as it is replaced by a new impression of an object. This process is repeated with increasing degrees of independence from the regressive conditions that were necessary to initiate the process of replacement. The structures of the grandiose self and ego ideal, which originally formed out of dependency and narcissistic need, gradually become increasingly object related and independent.

The Process of Replacement of the Representations of Infantile Objects

Each step in development is a more advanced expression of the steps that have preceded it. The system of object representations was founded upon the mental impressions of independent stimuli, which had the effect of evoking body ego experiences. The original model for this process was in the representation of the background object of primary identification, which established a foundation for the fusion and merger experiences of a psychological symbiosis. With advances in differentiation, the impressions of a separate object could be utilized to form mental structures that fostered self-expansion. Those impressions, which were based upon narcissistically determined attachments to an object, exert an influence that is in opposition to independent, autonomous, object-related functioning and now are in need of replacement. The grandiose self and the ego ideal are the remaining narcissistic structures that are accessible to the integrative functions of the ego.

In the pregenital phases of development, mental structures that united and differentiated the self- and object systems of representation utilized differing impressions of the same object. Although the impressions of a variety of external objects had an effect on the composition of these structures, the dominant effect was that of the primary object. With advances in development and the maturation of perceptual functions, there has been some degree of modification and freedom from the exclusiveness of the primary attachment. In addition, the process of depersonification of the fixation point on the projective arm of perception and integration of the fixation point on the introjective arm of perception have also loosened the ties to infantile experiences. There is thus a state of readiness to create a new version of the grandiose self and ego ideal that will be independent of these narcissistic influences.

The grandiose self is an instinctual structure, composed of the representation of good instinctual self-experience attached to the influence of a good instinctual object by the object's fantasy elaboration. It is formed during the anal phase to balance the experience of vulnerability with separateness, is based upon self-experiences of mastery and control, and is structurally linked by a fantasy of the object's omnipotence. This narcissistic attachment to the influence of a good instinctual object can only be replaced by creating a new interaction with a new independent object, which is capable of being represented as a replacement. The new interaction must be evocative of the original conditions of vulnerability and need for a good instinctual object's influence.

The establishment of a genital organization responsive to the increase in instinctual demand, ushering in the pubescent period, motivates the search for new independent love objects. The experience of crushes reflects the initiation of this process of replacing the infantile instinctual attachment at the foundation of the grandiose self. A crush, in pubescence, involves the representation of good genital instinctual self-experience attached to the fantasy of a good independent instinctual object's influence. The initial condition that must be fulfilled is that the interaction replicate the original narcissistic attachment, and it can then be represented in the structural position of the original object. The grandiose self originally formed during a critical period of development, to compensate for the experience of vulnerability by participating in a good instinctual object's omnipotence. The new edition of the grandiose self is also formed during a critical period of development, to compensate for the experience of vulnerability by participating in a fantasy of a good instinctual object's influence. The new attachment is object related, and the vulnerability is associated with genital instinctual experience. It is an instinctual attachment and is the first of numerous gradual steps toward attaining freedom from the need for resonance with the primary attachment and disengagement from its influence.

The ego ideal is a structure based upon selective identifications, composed of the representation of self-potentials elaborated in fantasy, and attached to the impressions of an object that is needed and admired. In this way, the influences of an object are included within self-experience to strengthen adaptive and integrative capacites. In the pregenital phases of development, the impressions of an object most admired were narcissistically determined. With the resolution of the oedipal conflict, selective identifications become increasingly object related. The original narcissistic attachment, embodied in the ego ideal, exerts its effect by maintaining the infantile object as a source of identification. The replacement takes place as new objects are selected as heroes to worship and as the impressions of these new experiences are available for identifications. These identifications occur from the perspective created by an object-related view of the new object and initially are resonant with identifications from a narcissistic orientation. Increasing exposure to the integrative effects of object-related, reality-oriented perceptions discriminates and disengages the representations of new objects from their infantile counterparts.

Falling in love leads to the replacement of the infantile instinctual attachment to an object comprising the grandiose self. The selection of heroes and ideals leads to the replacement of the narcissistically determined identifications with an object that comprise the ego ideal. Through a process of succeeding replacements, an increasing independence from the influence of these infantile attachments evolves. The original structures then occupy a place in the organization of an ever-expanding id of the dynamic unconscious, continue to serve a regulating function, maintain the boundary of the preconscious system, and participate in the formation of derivatives that give expression to unconscious mental content.

The Readiness for Genital Discharge: A Structured, Regulated Pathway for Instinctual Integration

The continuity of instinctual experience is represented within good self-experience as phase-specific instinctual gratification, shades into an aspect of bad self-experience as defenses are instituted, and extends to the impression of an overstimulating instinctual object. This continuity of experience outlines a pathway from instinctual activity that has been potentially traumatic at the interior, to instinctual activity that has attained sublimation and secondary autonomy at the periphery. In the absence of a structure uniting the portal of entry of instinctual demand to the system of self-representations, this pathway is tenuous and unreliable.

Instinctual representation achieves the limits of its expansion, within a narcissistically organized personality, with the evolution of the component instincts. Further progression requires an ever-increasing inclusion and integration of expanding dimensions of biophysiological demand, which depends upon the development of a capacity for object-related perceptions and experiences. The continuum of biophysiologic demand possesses an unseen dimension, which, in a narcissistic organization, is registered as an ominous, instinctual presence that is traumatic. A stable, regulated, and structured pathway of instinctual integration necessitates an ability to perceive an object as having unseen instinctual qualities. Without this perceptual capacity, the only alternative is to vigorously defend against including this aspect on the continuum of instinctual demand within the realm of mental representation.

During the phallic phase of psychosexual development, a shift, from a narcissistic to an object-related orientation, begins to take place. A fixation point is formed on the introjective arm of perception, which creates sufficient stability for the genital instinctual fantasies of the oedipal conflict to flourish. These genital fantasies, of bad self-experience and of a bad object's influence, provide the linkages that are structured to ensure cohesiveness at the interior and enable object-related perceptions to become functional and nontraumatic. An object-related perception registers body ego experiences in response to the recognition of an object's having unseen objects of its own and an independent instinctual life. It also registers the unseen dimension on the continuum of biophysiologic demand and includes it within the self-experience. Genitally determined primal scene fantasies (elaborated from the impression of a bad overstimulating instinctual object) are structurally linked to the representations of bad instinctual self-experience to establish a continuous, uninterrupted influx of instinctual demand. Once instinctual activity has access to representation within self-experience, the potential is present for exposure to the integrative processes that lead to sublimation and secondary autonomy.

At the same time that an instinctual pathway of integration is structured by primal scene fantasies, a second defense, consolidating new instinctual structure, is also formed. This structure creates a new object-related boundary for the unconscious system, by linking the incestuous fantasies elaborated from the representations of bad genital instinctual experience to the impressions of an overstimulating object. The prohibitive influences of an object tend to be mobilized in response to this union, which aids in the task of regulation. This structure has no perceptual function but is responsive to the effects of unconscious mental activity by eliciting appropriate derivatives. A reliable flow of instinctual activity, from its portal of entry to inclusion with self-experience, requires the establishment of a solid, flexible boundary to delineate the unconscious system. In the pregenital, narcissistic phases of development, the boundary was maintained by impingements and the reactions to them. This was a rigid, nondiscriminatory boundary that limited the extent to which instinctual activity could be represented.

The final step on the pathway of instinctual integration involves the process of including genital experiences of overstimulation within the realm of self-experience that does not require defense. The selective identifications motivated by the oedipal conflict strengthen good self-experience and enable this transition. This movement is associated with a dissolution of the fixation point on the introjective arm of perception. During the period of oedipal organization, this fixation point functioned to stabilize perceptual experience. Every stimulus, whether it emanated from the internal or external worlds, was perceived as having qualities determined by the memory traces of instinctual experience embodied in the fixation point. When a genital organization is structured, it serves as an obstacle to new experience and must be relinquished. At that point, the pathway of instinctual integration is complete, and the regulatory forces in the personality are consolidating to prepare for the impact of genital discharge.

The evolution of varied systems of consciousness, with well-defined boundaries and regulatory principles, is an integral aspect of maintaining a flow of instinctual activity. It allows instinctual demands to be represented in differing sectors of the personality, with varying degrees of neutralized energy. The superego monitors the movement of instinctual activity on its passage toward attaining full integration, which will ultimately be the pathway of genital discharge. The outcome of the formation and resolution of an oedipal conflict is the establishment of a structured pathway for instinctual integration and an independently functioning superego. When the superego functions of prohibition, regulation, guidance, and self-observation are in harmony with the interests of the ego, it is indicative of a readiness for selecting new love objects. It also reflects the presence of a structured, well-regulated pathway for instinctual integration and a readiness for genital discharge.

The Relationship of the Fixation Points to the Conflict-Free Sphere

The sudden increase in genital instinctual demand and the profound bodily changes that accompany it make pubescence and adolescence a crucial developmental period. The conditions and opportunities are present for replacing the representations of primary infantile attachments to an object and for a gaining an autonomous, independent, object-related existence. The individual's attitude toward the life experiences of love, work, and play can then facilitate the full realization of self-potentials, and there is sufficient autonomy and independence for the tasks necessary to sustain these experiences to be self-enhancing. The alterations in the fixation points, which took place in latency, have prepared the way for the evolution of a genital character and enabled this approach to become viable. A genitally organized character offers the necessary background of support to engage in experiences, selectively chosen, with the guidance and regulation of reality-oriented, conflict-free forces within the personality.

The conflict-free sphere has required the formation of boundaries to define it as a consolidated system of mental functions. It began to emerge as an organized system at the point in development when the oedipal situation was unfolding. Previously, conflict-free autonomous ego functions either operated in isolation or were utilized in the formation of perceptual boundaries during the narcissistic stages of self-expansion. The conflict-free sphere has been organizing at the point of perceptual contact with the external world. Its outer boundary is composed of the representations of empathic interactions with the primary object, which have occurred from an object-related perspective and have been conflict free. They reflect the experience of a separate good object's in-

fluence that has transpired under conditions in which differentiation has been well established. The fixation point on the projective
arm of perception was originally formed to stabilize the recognition of a separate good object's influence and necessitated the inclusion of its bad qualities due to the primitive level of
differentiation. This point of fixation must be maintained to anchor object constancy and to serve as a background for the effective functioning of projective mechanisms. Both the outer
boundary of the conflict-free sphere and the fixation point on the
projective arm of perception are based on the perception of a separate good object's influence. One is the memory trace of an infantile narcissistic attachment incorporating good and bad anal
qualities; the other is a more independent, autonomous, and
object-related attachment. The outer boundary of the conflict-free
sphere is exposed to the maturing functions of the ego and is
elaborated into depersonified symbolic and ideational expressions
of the attachment to an independent object. The eye of consciousness registers the evocative connection to a good object's influence
that is incorporated in the fixation point on the projective arm of
perception, which is then expanded by the addition of the depersonified contents of the conflict-free sphere. This process of depersonification, which is initiated in latency and continues
throughout the life cycle, maintains a fixation point on the projective arm of perception that has gained increasing independence
from the influences of the original infantile attachment. It is continuously expanded by the depersonified representations of object-
related attachments, which are essential for the processes of
thought, language, and symbolization to flourish.

The introjective arm of perception must remain open and be
relatively free of memory, for new experiences to be registered.
In the course of early pregenital development, it had to remain
open for new body ego experiences and object impressions to be
internalized. These were represented to build the structures necessary to shift from a narcissistic to an object-related orientation.
The introjective arm of perception was fixated during the oedipal
period to provide the stability for new structures to develop that
enabled an object-related perception of the inner and outer worlds.
The fixation point then had to be integrated and relinquished to
facilitate the internalization of new object-related experiences. In-

stinctual demand, which has traversed a structured pathway of integration and attained secondary autonomy, is represented and available to form the interior border of the conflict-free sphere. The final step in this pathway of instinctual integration is the dissolution of the fixation point on the introjective arm of perception. New experiences are narcissistically determined during the pregenital phases of development. The establishment of object-related perceptions and the changes in the fixation points have made it possible to perceive the similarities and differences in varying objects that include their independent qualities. Within a genital organization, a given stimulus can be registered in the varying systems of consciousness, simultaneously.

Pubescence: A New Period of Separation–Individuation

The psychological changes of pubescence are initiated in the male with the first ejaculatory experience, and in the female with the onset of the menarche. In the male, the anxiety associated with genital discharge is an indicator of the need to more effectively integrate instinctual activity. In the female, the anxiety associated with the first menstruation is an indicator of the need to more solidly establish feminine identifications. In order to accomplish these developmental tasks, there is a need in both to replace the infantile attachments to objects that are incorporated in the structure of the grandiose self and ego ideal. In this sense, pubescence introduces a new period of separation–individuation.

The initial period of separation–individuation took place when perceptual processes were immature, differentiation was unstable, and experiences were narcissistically determined. The representation of those infantile attachments remain, and the pubescent period is occupied with disengaging from their influence. This new separation–individuation phase takes place when perceptual processes have matured, differentiation is well established, and experiences are object related. The developmental task of pubescence and adolescence is successfully negotiated when the representations of infantile attachments, included in the grandiose self and ego ideal, are replaced. As a consequence, there is a change in orientation, so that the self is enhanced through interest in the object. Under the influence of narcissistic attachments, the object only has meaning in relation to what it provides.

The first experiences of falling in love are a manifestation of the representation of a new love object's occupying the position previously held by the representation of an infantile object. These experiences often seem regressive in nature, but they can be more appropriately referred to as a regression in the service of development. Falling in love reflects the replacement of the infantile object embodied in the grandiose self, whereas involvement with new heroes reflects the replacement of the infantile objects that structure the ego ideal. The focus of attention is upon the object, and the self is enhanced by the experience. The question is no longer, "Does the object love me?" The statement now is, "I am enhanced by virtue of experiencing love for the object." Self-esteem is no longer so dependent upon the responses of an external object but is determined by the realization of self-potentials and the ability to be involved with an object.

Discussion

On those occasions when a given function is transiently lost and then regained over a relatively short span of time, the underlying structures that determine the function become more clearly discernible. Within the contained and containing conditions of the therapeutic interaction, A had demonstrated the functional activities of self-observation, introspection, instinctual integration, and a continuing expansion in his capacity to represent psychic experience. A was confronted with the impact of an "accident" just prior to his session. The unconscious forces that dictated the accident, combined with an unempathic impinging external response, resulted in a transient loss of these advanced psychic functions. A's adaptive response was determined by regressive mental structures, and he was in a state of panic. He felt driven to seek reinforcement for the unstable defensive organization that was in the ascendancy.

The therapist's intervention had a containing influence, and a more advanced ego organization was gradually reestablished. The functions of self-observation and inner regulation became available; this was manifested in *A*'s ability to perceive the eruption of primitive aggression and the mobilization of a harsh, punitive defensive response. *A* stated that it felt as though his whole life had passed before his eyes—the later aspects first, and the earlier aspects later. When he first arrived at his session, the regressive threat of fragmentation had elicited an inner demand to contact his mother. He recognized the latent presence of a capacity to reestablish more advanced developmental structures. This was expressed in his feeling that if he could hold on to his perception of the experience, he would not feel panic.

A talked, anxiety was relieved, psychic functions gradually reemerged, and he became involved in a process of inner exploration and introspection. This seemed to be a reflection of his identification with a therapeutic attitude that had become structuralized. *A*'s comment that the first thing you lose is the last thing you get expressed his awareness that the integrative effects of self-observation was a new acquisition. The infantile attachment to an object, incorporated in the structure of the ego ideal, had been replaced by the representation of a new object. This underlying structure had stabilized the function of self-observation, which had been transiently lost in response to the stress evoked by the accident. The therapist's intervention elicited the activity of this later psychic acquisition, making it viable and functional.

Evidence of available structure remained, even in the presence of a regressive breakdown in function. *A*'s thought that the car looked like his mother's car was a derivative expression of unconscious mental activity. The ability to form derivatives is indicative of a psychic organization capable of continuity of experience and of some measure of containment. This was temporarily lost as the available structures were unable to contain the intensity of the demand, and there was a sudden shift into an action discharge mode of expression. The aggressive action immediately mobilized the primitive representation of a severely impinging and attacking object. *A*'s reaction was to seek out the therapist, indicating the latent viability of his attachment to the process of inner exploration. Simultaneously, he sought reassurance to alleviate his fragmentation anxiety. In the earlier stages of *A*'s psychotherapy, the therapist had offered containment to buffer the impact of narcissistic injuries and overstimulation. The representation of these experiences had established a foundation for negotiating the process of separation–individuation. At this later stage, the narcissistic infantile attachments had been largely replaced by new object-related attachments, though they were readily evoked under conditions of stress. A's desperate cry to reach his mother was motivated by this infantile attachment, and his response to the therapist's interpretive intervention was based upon a new object-related attachment. The process of replacing an infantile narcissistic representation of the therapist with a new object-related representation was reminiscent of the new period of separation–individuation associated with pubescence.

L was a child, in the midst of his pubescent period, who displayed an intermingling of healthy and pathological processes. Phobic symptomatology and a narcissistic manner of perceiving stimuli were manifestations of the pathological forces that influenced his functioning. His fear of the monster in the closet was expressive of a phobic attachment to the representation of an infantile object, whereas the hero worship of his piano and Hebrew teachers was indicative of an attempt at replacement with a new object. L sought the qualities of optimal gratification, autonomy, and uniqueness that were embodied in his perception of these figures. The story, told to him by his mother, captured the essence of the varied ways in which he was influenced by his infantile attachments. One aspect involved his enormous need for being special and unique, as he was to his mother during his early oral period. Another aspect concerned his struggle with injustice and fight for autonomy and separateness. L admired, respected, and feared his father, who served as a source of identification and as a source of severe prohibitive responses to instinctual overstimulation. The elements of hero worship were modeled by the identifications with his father and shaped by the experience of specialness in his early attachment to the mother.

The initial identifications with the therapist were resonant with, and paralleled, these infantile representations. The therapeutic relationship intensified, and the associated identifications attained increasing independence from this narcissistic influence. One consequence was in projective mechanisms and ideational activity's becoming more functional, as the underlying structure of the ego ideal provided a more stable background. L described the relief he experienced with the newfound ability to think. He was increasingly able to be introspective, and an expanded capacity for instinctual representation was manifested in the proliferation of derivatives. *L* then developed a crush, which reflected his first experience of replacing an instinctual attachment to an infantile object with a new object. This love relationship was a derivative expression of his feeling of closeness to the therapist.

L illustrated the significance of this new development in his descriptions of the relationship. He valued it highly, though the loved figure was far away and to a large extent unattainable. However, he felt connected by a bond of empathic resonance that made the distance tolerable. The anxiety he felt with the depth of the attachment involved being hurt and rejected, which was an expression of the influence of his original infantile instinctual attachment. The developmental thrust of pubescence to form instinctual attachments to new independent objects was observable. Initially, the experience with a new object was parallel to the regressive conditions of the original instinctual attachment. The difference was determined by the shift that had transpired, from a narcissistic orientation that is associated with infantile objects to an object-related orientation that is associated with a new independent object. *L's* anticipated fears were thus of narcissistic concerns of hurt and rejection, but he felt fulfilled from the experience of feeling love for the object. The therapist's interpretation of the transferential significance of *L's* love relationship was followed by an expanded awareness of the effects of developmental experiences upon his ability to love, and upon his defensive reactions. *L* then remarked that, as difficult as the experience was, he still valued it highly. His new love relationship had gained an increasing independence from the influence of the primary infantile attachment.

In *A* and *L*, a regressive, defensive, narcissistic orientation dominated the manner in which the stimuli of the internal and external worlds were perceived. Both had formed the new structures necessary for the perception of object-related experiences but had regressed to an earlier narcissistic organization. In *A* the regression was precipitated by stress, on a background of severe early pathology. In *L* the regression was a manifestation of his existing character pathology. In both, narcissistically determined infantile attachments to an object exerted an influence upon the therapeutic relationship. *A* readily reinstituted the functioning of structures based upon new object-related attachments, and *L* reenacted a new process of separation and individuation with the therapist.

The importance of self-observation in facilitating instinctual integration was apparent in both *A* and *L*. When *A* was under stress, this function was temporarily lost, and the perceptual activity of a poorly stabilized superego eye assumed dominance. The reestablishment of self-observation was accompanied by an alleviation of his fragmentation anxiety and an enlarged capacity to integrate instinctual activity. *L*'s difficulty in regulating instinctual demands was diminished in direct proportion to his rising ability to be introspective.

The differences in perceptual experience when the fixation point on the introjective arm of perception is closed and when it is open were evidenced in *A*'s perception of the accident. Under stress, he had regressed to an earlier position in which all stimuli were perceived in a fixed manner. The accident and all external objects were perceived as extensions of the internal objects that were attacking him. As more advanced psychic structures became functional, the fixation point on the introjective arm of perception was open to new experiences. *A* then perceived the accident in differing ways, at differing levels of organization. He perceived it as a new experience, and, simultaneously, he perceived the unique and individual meaning that it evoked within him. The psychological changes associated with pubescence were occurring in *A* well beyond the time of his physiological pubescence. The severity of his pathology had not allowed the psychic changes of pubescence to occur at the time that genital discharge was first manifested. The process of replacing the attachments to infantile objects, with new independent objects, had to be delayed.

CHAPTER 11

The Final Step to Maturity
The Genital Character

Introduction

The complexities of human psychological development are such that any given individual manifests varying admixtures of healthy and pathological forces. The interweaving of a multiplicity of influences shapes the personality, until an overall predominant mode of adapting and responding to stimuli emerges. In the preceding chapters, the central focus has been on illuminating those ingredients that, when continuously present, eventuate in a healthy functioning human being. An attempt has been made to integrate the insights of instinctual theory, object relations theory, and a psychology of the self from an ego psychological point of view, by emphasizing the role of perception. The foundation for continuing the progression of healthy development, throughout the life cycle, depends upon the formation of a genitally organized character structure.

A *genital character* can be defined by the manner in which the major experiences of work, play, and love are selected and are included in an individual's life. Each of these experiences requires the smooth and harmonious functioning of all psychic processes and adaptational mechanisms in order to be fully realized. Although there is some overlapping, differing psychic structures are highlighted in response to the unique and individual significance of each of these life processes. A hallmark of the genital character is the selection of love relationships, play activities, and work

313

situations that express all dimensions of the personality, are balanced in their proportions, and enhance the continuation of self-expansion.

The process of work highlights the functioning of the superego. In the genital character, instinctual activity is granted expression through an integrated pathway. Superego responses are regulatory and guiding, rather than prohibitive, and gentle restraint is the predominant inhibitory force. The individual's work performance and achievements are not experienced as proof of strength or power but do provide narcissistic gratification. These narcissistic elements are not compensatory in nature and include involvement with an object. The ego ideal, based on selective identifications with new and independent objects, is guided by the participation of the conflict-free sphere. Realizable self-potentials are in close approximation to the fantasy elaborations utilized in establishing these identifications.

The process of play highlights the functioning of the ego. In the genital character, instinctual demand is well regulated and granted sublimatory expression without the need for excessive restraints. The pregenital component instincts, invested with differing degress of neutralized energy, are allowed gratification under selected conditions. Aggression is differentiating in its effects, fuels self-assertiveness, and enables realistic actions in the external world. Actions and affective experiences are intense and spontaneous, and there is ample energy for adaptive defensive responses that are flexible and well controlled. The genital character can be joyful, but also angry, experience loss with depression and not be enveloped by it, love intensely, hate intensely, and be childlike without being infantile. The expression of courage is present, not to compensate for deficiencies, but to attain a given goal. Seriousness is natural with an openness to the external world that can be as intense in one situation as the ability to shut off the impact of the external world is in another. In the genital sexual act with a loved partner, the ego can be reduced to the function of perception as the individual is engulfed by pleasure without anxiety or the need for excessive defense. Relationships with the external world are based upon a realistic orientation guided by the participation of an organized system of conflict-free ego functions.

The process of love highlights the functioning of the id. In the genital character, love relationships are genitally determined and are relatively free of ambivalence. The incestuous and rivalrous strivings, associated with the oedipal conflict, no longer direct object-seeking behavior. Genital interest is in new heterosexual objects that no longer are representations of infantile instinctual objects. The oedipal conflict has served its organizing function, and pregenital instinctual demands are sublimated and gratified in the act of forepleasure. Genital primacy is well established as the sexual act itself offers the greatest pleasure and is the most important sexual goal.

In this chapter, I will present an overview of the pregenital attachments to an object that must be replaced in order to attain a genitally organized character. I will also describe the processes of work, play, and love, and the importance of the activities that sustain them.

Clinical Material

In *A*'s final year of high school, his thoughts of graduation were associated with the termination of his therapy. They both represented a time for him to establish an independent existence. He felt it was the right time to be leaving therapy. His mind was constantly occupied with his life goals—what he wanted and how he could attain it. He selected a date for ending his therapy that would not coincide with the therapist's vacation or with his graduation from school. He wanted it to stand by itself. As the date approached, he spent many of his sessions reviewing experiences with the therapist. He took special delight in recalling the therapist's mistakes and in chiding the therapist for his blindness and stupidity. He occasionally became serious when he remembered how cut off he felt from all human contact and the impact it had upon him when the therapist found a way to reach him. The following session occurred several weeks prior to his final day.

A began talking about his mounting anxiety as graduation from school came nearer. His life in school was so defined and structured. He ruminated as to what he would do without it. The therapist stated that he was reminded of the times when *A* had been concerned as to the solidity of the therapist's image inside of him. Perhaps he was now worried about his ability to carry this with him when therapy ended. *A* was silent and remembered when he had called from the airport. "That was such a long time ago." It seemed funny to him now. *A* then spoke of what he wanted to do. He wanted to join the military service, especially the marines. "They make a man out of you." He went on to describe how much he liked the idea; he could be on his own, but there would be a lot around him. He would not have to worry about where to live and how he would get meals. He would be on his own, and yet have confidence that the things surrounding him were taken care of. *A* felt he needed that until he could feel more confident about managing it himself. He could also learn to fight. He would not have to fight, but he would know how. He began to animatedly fantasy himself fighting. He then paused and went on to talk of his wish to enlist. He could feel, like he belonged to something important. His parents opposed the idea. They kept telling him it would be too much, or too demanding, or that he would not be strong enough. They repetitively told him how unrealistic he was in considering it. They put special emphasis on his medical history and told him it would prevent him from being accepted. *A* paused and looked at the therapist, "Would that keep me out?" The therapist commented that *A* seemed to be asking if the therpaist was worried about his ability to be separate and independent. *A* spoke of how right it felt to him. His mother was always fearful of every decision he made. He firmly stated, "I can't make my mother's fears mine." He went on to describe how uneasy he felt whenever his mother was fearful. It was as though he took her feeling into himself. *A* then elaborated on the efforts he had been making to get information about the military. He planned to enlist prior to his graduation, so that he would have a direction.

M was a 6-year-old boy, referred in response to his school's concern over his isolated and withdrawn behaviors. His parents saw him as an extremely independent child. They were at times worried about his intense determination to accomplish tasks beyond his abilities, and they were surprised at the depth of the school's concern. When he came to his first session, *M* was fearful, embarrassed, and clung to his mother. This was surprising to the mother, as *M* had never exhibited this behavior before. He stated that he could not talk, but his body could. When the therapist remarked that he would try to understand his body's messages, *M* immediately came into the office. He drew a picture that he called his fort. It had no doors or windows, and he was perfectly safe where no one could hurt him. The therapist reflected upon the great expense *M* seemed to pay for his safety; nothing could come in, and he was limited in not being able to get out. *M* commented that he could find a way out if he wanted to. He later agreed with the therapist that it would be a good idea to meet regularly and explore whether he would want to find a way out.

During the early months, *M* vacillated between laboriously working on some project that he brought in and being teasing and provocative. He gradually revealed how tightly controlled his emotions were and how frightened he was of "letting go." Someone, including himself, would get hurt. He cautiously tested the therapist to determine if it was safe. On a few occasions, he brought ropes to tie up the therapist. He fantasied being in total control and having the freedom to ravage the office. The idea was extremely exciting to him. He "inadvertently" knocked over some object in the room and was immediately reminded of people who were weak and helpless and for whom he felt contempt. The therapist's comment that *M* seemed to be coming out of his fort and was fearful that the therapist would be helpless in containing him especially when he could so easily knock over his belongings was facilitating to *M*. He laughed and drew a picture of the fort, indicating that construction work was being done on the doors and windows. The following session took place shortly after *M* had developed a vivid fantasy of his mother's being in total despair and attempting to kill herself by jumping out of a window. She was rescued by *M*, who stopped her at the very last moment.

M entered the office, appearing wild and uncontrollable. He began to yell and race around the room in an overexcited fashion. He grabbed an object and threw it across the room. The therapist held him gently, and *M* began to protest, rapidly coming to the point of tears. "Don't trap me. You're hurting my feelings." When released, he once again became wild and excited. The therapist again held him; this time stating that *M* had the key to be free. *M* became wild and excited; the therapist held him; *M* indicated that he wanted to be released, and he was free. This behavior continued for a time. With great surprise, M exclaimed, "I'm playing." He went on to refer to his inability to pretend. He could imagine things, but he could not play. The therapist wondered if anything came into M's mind that could show what he was playing. M became thoughtful and then wanted to use the therapist's furniture to play a game. He constructed a den, which he crawled into through a small opening. He crawled inside and began to coo like a baby. It was warm and comfortable inside his den; he could be a baby. The opening was so small; he felt like it might suffocate him to crawl out. He giggled as he reveled in being a baby.

N, a woman in her early 30s, was in the process of obtaining a divorce from her second husband. She had great difficulty in managing her life and was frightened that she was going to kill herself. She had been on the verge of doing so when she called for an appointment. During the early phases of therapeutic contact, secrets were highlighted. Every session was occupied with the revelation of a new secret. They all involved relationships that she had kept secret. Many were of intense and brief sexual encounters, with N submitting to the wishes of her partner. She feared the therapist would see her as bad and promiscuous. Another secret concerned her two marriages. The first occurred at age 18, when she was seeking a way to escape home. She married a young man who lived with his mother, moved from her home to his, and felt trapped. She was too dependent and felt she was being destroyed by her need to be taken care of. She made an effort to go to school, learned a trade, got divorced, and attempted to live on her own. The secret of this marriage was of her dependence. The therapist would think of her as bad in marrying someone she did not love. The second marriage was to a man she saw as extremely exciting. He lived on the edge of danger at all times. She helped him in his work, found it exciting, and at first felt free. Gradually, she began to feel engulfed and overwhelmed by her second husband's jealousy and possessiveness. She was attracted to his father, felt like a small child when in his presence, and at first perceived him as warm and caring. Later, as she knew him better, he appeared aloof and distant. She realized her illusions had created this image and was frightened that she could not trust her own perceptions. She became increasingly terrified of her second husband and began to feel that her life was in danger. She feared leaving him because any move in that direction precipitated an intense jealous rage. She felt ashamed of her participation in this relationship and of revealing it to the therapist. Although N had managed to complete school in order to develop an independent existence, she now felt as though all of her efforts led to nothing. Her love relationships were all destructive, and she felt she had no reason to live. Her child was the one thread that held her to living, and she even questioned that.

There were also secrets that emerged from her genetic past. She was the oldest of three children and discovered her mother had a sexual liason with another man while married to her father and that this man was her biologic father. She had always been teased about not looking like others in the family. She was with her mother when they met a man who had children resembling her. The mother threatened her with keeping this meeting a secret. A second secret occurred earlier in her life. Her grandfather was a well-respected pharmacist in a small town. The patient spent time in his store and noticed her grandfather disappear for periods of time. She explored and found him masturbating to pornographic pictures. She was also threatened with keeping this discovery a secret.

The need for an ongoing therapeutic interaction was identified early in the first hour, and the framework and ground rules were established during the early sessions. Discussion focused upon the fee, the times, and the frequency. N described herself as having very little money. She was attempting to raise a family on her own, received little child support, and was in the first stages of a divorce. In addition, she did not want third-party involvements, such as insurance. She was fearful that her husband would discover she was seeing a psychiatrist and use it as evidence to take her child away. For the same reason, she did not want a bill and did not want to pay by check. Her associations to the fee were of situations when people had done her favors and it had always turned out badly; there was either an ulterior motive, or it was infantilizing. The therapist responded by stating that he thought N was showing him how essential it was for her to pay a full fee, and this was agreed upon. N seemed to be describing the ideal conditions of a therapeutic framework but was consciously using all of the wrong reasons. The therapist felt it reflected an unconscious awareness of the well-contained framework she would need for therapy to be successful. It appeared to express how poorly contained she felt during her developmental years and offered a guide for the conduct of her sessions.

Throughout the course of N's therapy, it was essential that the framework and ground rules be solidly maintained, clear-cut, and not yield to the pressures she exerted to disrupt it. The therapist was experienced as a good object when he offered interpretations of her efforts to alter the frame. This helped N to see herself (and was optimally gratifying), amplified functions so that she experienced her inner resources (and was optimally frustrating), and gave her the psychological space to experience the therapist in whatever way was important to her (the qualities of a transitional object). She alternately thought of the therapist as a prostitute, as an authority who disapproved of her, or as someone aroused by her. N frequently exerted pressure upon the therapist to not be so rigid and inflexible, to talk on the phone outside of the hours, or to change the hours to an earlier or later time. The reasons would involve seemingly unalterable realities—to better herself in her career, a work commitment, or an event associated with her child. The therapist's attitude remained constant. He encouraged N to associate and interpreted her efforts to gain defensive reinforcement and negate the therapist as a good object. She occasionally succeeded in evoking an image in the therapist of himself as a cold, rigid, unfeeling person. On those occasions, N would be filled with the feeling that she was bad and destructive, and this made anyone close to her equally bad. These moments were interpreted as her unconscious perception of the therapist's wavering in response to her pressure. The following session occurred after a sequence of hours in which N felt contained and recognized the value of the therapist's position.

N came in crying. She felt lost, confused, and paralyzed. She feared she was losing an important relationship with a loved figure in her life. She felt the need to cling to him but also felt that everything was unreal and that she was being swallowed up. N sobbed deeply as she talked of falling into a pit, feeling trapped, and like she wanted to die. The therapist stated that as N felt contained, she could allow the inner objects that occupied her mind to come closer to her. This created a feeling of being engulfed and enveloped by their presence. She felt the urge to cling to old defensive ways and could not. N silently cried and remembered seeing a young girl at a bus stop. It was winter, the girl was alone and cold, and N wanted to comfort her. It made her feel so sad. She then recalled shopping with her daughter. N had picked out a dress for her daughter, who became enraged as she wanted to pick out her own. N then realized it was important to encourage her daughter's independence. She had always tried to do everything for her child so she would suffer no pain. She could see now that this attitude had hurt her daughter because she needed to be separate and be her own person. N returned to the love relationship she was losing. She felt enveloped by a state of mind with no perspective. How could she gain perspective? She paused, ''I know how. I can't have you be my mirror all of the time. I have to stand aside and look at myself.'' N imagined herself looking in a mirror. The image in the mirror was herself reflecting back what she saw. She saw herself as struggling to survive and perceived her feelings, not as evidence of badness but as a way of understanding her internal life.

The Pregenital Attachments to an Object and the Conditions Necessary for Their Replacement

The perceptual processes activate the representatonal and organizational functions of the ego, during the earliest phases of development, to create two realms of mental experiences. Body ego experiences are consolidated into a system of self-representations and their object-impression counterparts into a system of object representations. The two realms are first connected with the recognition of a separate good object's influence, which is stabilized by an awareness of its bad qualities. Fantasies are elaborated, within each realm of experience, which function to link the mental representations in one system to the mental representations in the other. Specific linkages are structured in response to the existing narcissistic conditions, which further unite and differentiate the two systems of representation. These initial stages of cohesiveness establish a foundation for continuing progression toward a genital organization and are based upon the representations of pregenital attachments to an object.

The grandiose self structurally unites the self-system with the object system to balance the experience of vulnerability with separateness during the anal phase, by participating in a fantasy of the object's omnipotence. The ego ideal structurally unites the object system with the self-system to strengthen adaptive capacities, by including admired qualities of an object's influence within self-experience. These structures are an integral part of the consolidation of the superego and are essential for the formation and resolution of an oedipal conflict. The resulting genital organization, accompanied by the emergence of object-related perceptions and object-related experiences, has advanced to the point where further progression necessitates independence from the influence that pregenital attachments continue to exert. The major task of pubescence and adolescence is to replace the original representations of infantile, pregenital attachments to an object that comprise the structures of the grandiose self and ego ideal. This developmental step must be negotiated to attain a genital sexual relationship with an independent love object. It is also necessary for the selection, guidance, and regulation of actions that enhance self-expansion to be unencumbered from the limitations imposed by these narcissistic influences.

During the pregenital stages of psychosexual development, there is a narcissistic orientation to all stimuli, and the perception of an object's having unseen independent objects is traumatic. The emergence and flourishing of an oedipal conflict serve as a psychic organizer, which instigates a shift to an object-related orientation. The oedipal conflict consists of the fantasies elaborated from the representation of genital instinctual self-experiences of overstimulation and from the representation of a genitally overstimulating object. These fantasies form structured linkages, uniting the two systems of representations at the interior of the personality, that ensure cohesiveness and continuity of experience. Primal scene fantasies link the object system with the self-system to form a structured pathway of instinctual integration. Incestuous fantasies link the self-system with the object system to form a new boundary for unconscious mental activity. New defensive unions are also formed to aid in regulating the increase in instinctual activity. This genital organization enables the capacity for object-related perceptions, and the unseen aspects of instinctual demand can be represented and included within self-experience for the first time. The associated recognition of an object, having unseen independent objects, can evoke body ego expriences without trauma. The fixation points, which have been essential to achieve this level of organization, become an obstacle to any further progress and have to change. They have been founded upon the representation of a pregenital attachment to an object and upon the representation of pregenital instinctual experience. The process of altering the fixation points is also the onset of attaining advancing degrees of independence from the influence of narcissistically determined developmental experiences.

The depersonification of the fixation point, on the projective arm of perception, initiates the abatement of the influence exerted by an infantile, narcissistic attachment to an object. This fixation point embodies the representation of a tie to a separate good anal object, with an awareness of bad anal qualities. The inclusion of bad qualities was essential in this early stage of narcissism because the relative lack of differerentiation and predominance of fusion–merger experiences worked against the recognition of a separate good object's influence. The memory traces, forming the outer boundary of the conflict-free sphere, consist of the representations of empathic, object-related interactions. These representations of a separate, independent, good object's influence operate as a foundation for the production of symbolized expressions of ego interests. The eye of consciousness connnects these depersonified representations of a good object's influence to the fixation point on the projective arm of perception, which is thereby expanded and depersonified. Conceptual, symbolizing, and projective mechanisms function on this stable, object-related background to use neutralized energy in the mental activities of thinking and abstraction. Advances, in the process of depersonification, increase the degree of separation from the influence of the primary infantile attachment that originally established this fixation point.

The final step on the structured pathway of instinctual integration has resulted in a dissolution of the fixation point on the introjective arm of perception. The representations of self-experiences of phallic overstimulation, in no longer requiring defense, have attained secondary autonomy and form the inner boundary of the conflict-free sphere. The introjective arm of perception is open once again and can register new object-related experiences relatively free of narcissistically determined influences.

The alterations in the fixation points prepare the way for the impact of pubescence. The enormous increase in instinctual demand and the extensive bodily changes motivate the final developmental steps to maturity. These involve the replacement of infantile attachments to an object with the representations of attachments to new and independent objects.

Replacing the Infantile Representations of an Object

The focused areas of perceptual activity, incorporated in the structures of the grandiose self and ego ideal, form boundaries within which the superego consolidates into an independently functioning agency. The representations of infantile, narcissistic attachments to primary objects that comprise the grandiose self and ego ideal continue to exert an effect upon the functions of the superego. With the establishment of a genital organization and the capacity for genital discharge, a point is reached in adolescence where further self-expansion through object-related experiences depends upon the selection of new love objects that are independent of the primary objects. In order to accomplish this task, the influence of the infantile attachments is diminished and eliminated by a process of replacing them with the representations of new and independent attachments to an object.

In pubescence, the fixation point on the introjective arm of perception has been relinquished, and new object-related experiences can be registered and represented. When an interaction with a new object is evocative to, and parallel with, the representations of the original infantile attachments, it becomes possible to initiate the process of replacement. The body ego experience and object impression, elicited by the effect of the new object, are represented in apposition to the attachment to a primary object but with a measure of independence from its narcissistic influence. The repetition of this process gradually gains freedom from the need to replicate the original attachment and eventuates in its replacement.

(This process of replacement characterizes the manner in which structural change takes place, through the regressive transference interaction, in psychoanalytic treatment. The conditions of psychoanalysis are designed to create an interactional environment that allows this process of replacement to take place.)

The grandiose self is an instinctual structure and requires an instinctual interaction, which parallels the original representation, for the infantile object to be replaced. The guiding function of the superego motivates the individual to seek out those conditions and types of interactions that parallel the original infantile attachment, which reflects its continuing influence. Object-seeking behavior and adaptive functions may appear regressive, but these are an expression of progress and in the service of development. Recreating the necessary conditions requires the suspension of more advanced perceptual functions. The phrase, "love is blind," has reference to these phenomena, in which the reality-oriented, integrative function of the eye of consciousness is suspended in order to create the conditions that lead to a replacement of this infantile representation. Perceptual activity is transiently registered by the superego eye. Interactions are recreated with a new object and registered by perceptual activity that is dominated by the influence of narcissistically determined structures. The perceptual activity of the eye of consciousness is alternately suspended and reinstated, which is a more avanced expression of the manner in which the original recognition of separateness was lost and recaptured. The representation of the new, independent object eventually replaces the infantile representation, creating a grandiose self that is relatively free of narcissistic influences. The guiding function of the superego is then more effective in the selection of new love objects.

The ego ideal is a noninstinctual structure, and the infantile attachments upon which it is based are therefore not as tenacious. The narcissistically determined selective identifications at its foundation have been gradually modified during the period of oedipal organization. This structure, in maintaining more direct contact with the integrative forces in the conscious system, has attained increasing independence from the influence of narcissistic attachments. The resolution of the oedipal conflict has resulted in selective identifications, along the pathway structured by the ego ideal, that are object-related in nature. During the pubescent and adolescent period, new object-related experiences are occurring with a multiplicity of external objects, concepts, and ideals. Initially, they are evocative of the object qualities included in the original identifications with the primary infantile object. These narcissistic representations are relatively readily replaced with the representations of new and independent objects. (This process of replacement is characteristic of the structural change that takes place, through identification with an analytic attitude, in psychoanalytic treatment.)

The replacement of the representations of primary infantile objects has facilitated a crucial change in perspective. Previously, it was the love and approval of the object that was essential, whereas now it is the ability to love and value the object that has become important. There is no longer a dependence upon external objects to elevate self-esteem. Self-esteem is regulated by the ability to be involved with, and love, an object. Disappointments, loss, rejections, and failures can be experienced for their unique individual meaning and not be experienced as depleting or damaging.

The Conflict-Free Sphere of Ego Functions in the Genital Character

The period of latency has often been referred to as a period of sexual quiescence. This does not mean that there is a diminution in instinctual demand or in instinctual activity. It has reference to the ascendency of integrative processes, to the changes in the fixation points, and to the increasing availability of ego functions that are free of conflict. These developments prepare for the major shifts that occur in pubescence and adolescence. The organization of a system of conflict-free ego functioning is of particular importance.

There is a difference between the presence of autonomous ego functions operating in isolation and a conflict-free system of ego functions. The autonomous ego functions are largely dependent upon the effects of maturation for their development and, in that sense, are objectless. However, for their full realization, there is a degree of dependence upon the amplifying responses of an empathic external object. This fosters a harmonious interrelationship between the autonomous ego functions and the representations of good self-experience and of a good object's influence. These ego functions are an integral part of the consolidation of self-experience into well-defined entities and are inextricably interwoven into the mental structures that unite and differentiate the self- and object systems of representation. They are in turn enhanced in their effectiveness as advancing levels of psychic organization are evolving.

The autonomous ego functions exert their activity at the point of perceptual contact with the external world. They are represented as a facet of good self-experience and thus begin to organize in close proximity to the area in which a fixation point is formed on the introjective arm of perception. The integration of this fixation point expands the range of activities that can utilize autonomous functions, with the added impetus of sublimated instinctual energies. The representations of phallic and genital instinctual experiences, which no longer require defense, have attained secondary autonomy and form an interior boundary for this organizing sphere of conflict-free ego activity. The fixation point on the introjective arm of perception formed to enable the structural foundation for a genital organization to develop. This took place at a time when the narcissistically determined needs for the empathic responses of the primary external object were fulfilled. With the shift to object relatedness, the awareness of the primary external object's independent instinctual life has a differentiating effect. Ongoing empathic interactions are represented from an object-related perspective and form an outer boundary for the conflict-free sphere. A conflict-free system of ego functioning is defined during the latency period and extends its sphere of influence with each step toward establishing a genital character. It is gradually integrated with the superego's guiding function in the choice of work situations, sublimatory play activities, and new love objects, and is also engaged with the process of depersonification that continues throughout the life cycle.

The system of conscious mental activity is ever expanding. The evolution of an organized system of conflict-free ego functioning, with boundaries and regulatory principles, is a significant aspect of that expansion. The projective arm of perception is extended and strengthened by its perceptual connection to the depersonified products of a good object's influence that are elaborated in the conflict-free sphere. This provides a foundation, supported by autonomous forces, that furthers processes of symbolization, language, and abstract thinking. Instinctual demand, having traversed a structured pathway of integration, is no longer bound to defensive responses, has attained secondary autonomy, and serves to continually enlarge the conflict-free sphere along its inner boundary. The dominant force in the personality has shifted, from the effects created by representations of early narcissistically determined developmental experience to the effects created by new object-related experiences. Self-enhancement and self-expansion are advanced through engagement in the major life experiences of work, play, and love, and in the activities that sustain them.

The Processes of Work, Play, and Love in the Genital Character and the Activities That Sustain Them

Work, play, love, and the activities that sustain them are major life experiences that give expression to the totality of the personality. In the genital character, they involve object-related interactions with the external world and are dependent upon a harmonious interplay of intrapsychic forces that include the participation of id, ego, and superego for effective functioning. Each of these life processes has a developmental line and highlights a particular aspect of the tripartite structures. Work emphasizes the functioning of the superego, although it requires the synchronous involvement of ego interests and functions and is motivated by sublimated id energies. Play underscores the functioning of the ego, although it requires the inclusion of instinctual id derivatives and the monitoring, regulating function of the superego. Love relationships are given their unique, individual meaning by the mental representations that occupy the id of the dynamic unconscious, although they necessitate the defensive and integrative functions of the ego and the guidance of the superego. Self-sustaining activities ensure the availability of these life experiences and are an integral aspect of self-realization. Self-care, exercise of responsibility, money management, awareness of time and space, and goal-directed behavior designed to provide opportunities are all examples of these activities. They are independent, autonomous actions that support and manage object-related, self-enhancing engagements with the external world and are evocative to the containing effects of the background object of primary identification.

Work incorporates ambitions and goals, which are directed by morals and standards, into the use of an individual's unique talents and skills. This process highlights the functioning of a well-integrated, independent superego agency, which facilitates the realization of ego interests with the aid of sublimated id energies. This definition coincides with Kohut's (1971) description of healthy narcissism. Kohut postulated a separate line of narcissistic development, in a bipolar self. Ambitions and goals expressed the mirroring pole; morals and standards expressed the idealizing pole; and the use of talents and skills an integration of the two. A bipolar self can be conceptualized in an entirely different manner that does not necessitate a separate line of narcissistic development. A bipolar self would then refer to the polarization of the self- and object systems of representation and the mental activities that are expressed in each locale. The representations of self-experience are at the foundation of instinctual activity and of introjective mechanisms. The representations of an object's influence are at the foundation of differentiating, restraining, regulatory activities, and of projective mechanisms. The use of talents and skills is the expression, in action, of the final step on a structured pathway of instinctual integration. Morals and standards are the manifestation of an integrated superego, achieved through selective identifications. Ambitions and goals reflect the interests of the ego in harmony with the guiding function of the superego. Work thus includes the participation of the id and ego but highlights the functioning of the superego.

Play includes masturbatory activities, the expression of the component instincts in the foreplay of a genital sexual love relationship, and the varied regressions in the service of the ego. It depends upon the availability and utilization of instinctual energies at differing levels of neutralization. The ego's resilient functioning is highlighted by the compromises that are effected in mobilizing mental structures that enable the expression of component instincts without full genital discharge. The superego continues to exert a regulatory, restraining function, and the contribution of the id is evident in the expression of the component instincts.

Love relationships are determined by a genital interest in new and independent external objects. The infantile attachments to primary objects have been replaced, and no longer play a role in the choice of a love object. However, the hierarchical organization of development experiences that occupy the id of the dynamic unconscious is actively evoked to give depth and individual meaning to love relationships. It is in this way that id functions are highlighted.

Self-sustaining activities can be experienced as enhancing, challenging, and fulfilling, or as depleting, demanding, and a source of resentment. When the processes of work, play, and love are a viable part of an individual's existence and are balanced in proportion, self-sustaining activities are enhancing and containing. These self-supportive actions are resonant with the background object of primary identification (represented as an aspect of good self-experience). It is usually an indication of stress and is often the first sign of psychological difficulty, when self-sustaining activities are experienced as drudgery or with resentment.

The nature of these life experiences is determined by the processes that are engaged in their realization. An individual's particular choice of occupation, for example, may be a self-sustaining activity and not involve the process of work. The "play" of a child is most frequently along the developmental line of work because the developmental line of play is associated with masturbatory activities and the various expressions of the component instincts. The varied ego functions utilized in self-care and the exercise of responsibility, when assumed in an age and phase-specific manner, are establishing a developmental line for their eventual independence in supporting work, play, and love relationships.

Discussion

The ability to distinguish healthy from pathological processes is essential for the conduct of an effective therapeutic interaction. When qualities are present that facilitate the ascendancy of healthy processes, they are unconsciously perceived and evoke derivatives expressive of the experience. Interpretive interventions that are empathically responsive to unconscious communications incorporate the combined qualities of a good object. These include optimal gratification, optimal frustration, and the qualities of a transitional object. *Optimal gratification* refers to the mastery, independence, autonomy, and self-regulation that are gained through insight and perspective; *optimal frustration* refers to the absence of collusion with pathological defenses, which have the effect of amplifying autonomous functions; and the *qualities of a transitional object* refers to the therapist's capacity to foster the patient's freedom to express the demands dictated by unconscious forces, within a contained, interpretive relationship. This framework is established, guided, and verified by the derivatives of unconscious perceptions. Pathological forces in the personality, based upon distortions and primarily adaptive to the stimuli of the internal world, can then become manifested and exposed to the integrative influences of healthy processes.

The establishment of a genital character signifies an ensured and effectively maintained structural foundation for continued growth and self-expansion through object-related experiences and is the equivalent of attaining the full realization of self-potentials. Within the personality of each individual, there is an interweaving of both healthy and pathological forces. In the fully formed genital character, the aspects reflective of pathology are transient, readily resolved, and offer no serious obstacle to continuing growth. Throughout this presentation, clinical examples of pathology have been utilized to explicate the characteristics and evolution of healthy psychological functioning. Even with a successful therapeutic outcome, the residuals of preexisting pathology are present within the personality and, under stress, will continue to exert an influence. A given individual is never entirely free of the multiple and complex interplay of forces that have shaped developmental experience.

A approached the termination of his therapy, and the ascendancy of healthy psychic functioning was observable. The continuing influence of the severe pathology that had dominated his early development was also evident. This clinical vignette illustrates the presence of a foundation for the processes of work to be realized and highlights the functioning of his superego. *A* had negotiated the shift from narcissism to object relatedness, although he continued to experience the effects of a relative instability in the structures that maintained cohesiveness and differentiation. When he was under stress, the influence of narcissistically determined structures was clearly present, but A could now rely upon inner regulation that was guided by an integrated and functional superego. A's choice of the military service as a work experience reflected the harmonious interplay between ego interests and the guiding function of the superego. It represented an opportunity for him to utilize his particular talents and skills in realizing ambitions and goals that were guided by morals and standards separate and independent of parental influences. This particular work choice was reminiscent of his earlier identifications with General Patton and his selection of football. The motive centered upon his search for a way to express aggression in a contained, regulated, and sublimated fashion. The continuing need for reinforcement of a relatively weak representation of the background object of primary identification was also involved in his work choice. He was attracted to an external environment in which support was ensured and secure.

A's reaction to his mother's anxiety and his question to the therapist concerning his medical history were indicative of the instability in his more advanced level of psychic organization. The residuals of earlier difficulties with separation–individuation continued to exert their effects. However, he responded to the therapist's interpretation by mobilizing his resources and displayed how readily an autonomous, independent position could resurface. A was engaged in selecting a work situation that was consonant with the realization of his potentials, independent of the influence of others, and that included his strengths and vulnerabilities. A genitally determined psychic organization was predominant, which gave expression to the ascendancy of healthy processes.

The processes of play highlight the functioning of the ego, as compromises are effected between the instinctual demands emanating from the id and the superego responses. Play activities are manifested in a fluid, harmonious, and spontaneous manner, with the ego's mediating intrapsychic experience utilizing varying levels of neutralized instinctual energy. M illustrated the effects of intense conflict upon his ability to effectively manage instinctual activity and a subsequent severe inhibition in the processes of play. He exhibited a fixed defensive response to all stimuli; this was expressed in descriptions of his fort. This was a place where he was perfectly safe but extremely limited in what he could take in or let out.

M was excessively overcontrolled and fearful of being controlled. The therapist's offer of an explorative relationship appeared to give M the feeling of being unconsciously understood, and he gradually revealed how fearful he was of emotions and their effect upon others. M, both behaviorally and through derivatives, expressed a wish to be contained and a fear of being trapped. The interpretation of his concern that the therapist would be helpless elicited a drawing in which his fort had doors and windows and then a fantasy of the despair of a mothering figure. M appeared to feel sufficiently contained to "let in" the therapist's words and to "let out" his feeling about a mother's helplessness. He then became alternately wild in his behavior and was crushed by the therapist's physical control. When the therapist put the control in M's hands, he felt comfortable and contained. He then noted with surprise that he was playing; that is, he was effecting the compromises characteristic of the process of play. The inhibition was alleviated, and M described his inability to play. He could form instinctual derivatives of unconscious mental activity (he could imagine), but he could not engage in actions that expressed the component instincts in a sublimated fashion (he could not play). The integrative effect of the therapeutic relationship, and the containment it offered, enabled M to act in ways that had previously been prohibited. His play, symbolizing the oral components of instinctual activity and the dangers associated with separation, required that his ego function to establish the necessary compromises.

N exemplified the profound influence that infantile attachments to an object can have upon the choice of new objects. Her selection of love objects was dictated by the conditions required by the representations of these infantile attachments. The particular pattern of her involvement with loved objects was in accordance with the narcissistically determined infantile experiences that dominated in her internal world. In her first marriage, she was attempting to escape the suffocating effects of oral dependency and was driven to select a relationship that recreated the conditions she was striving to escape. Her second marriage represented an attempt to realize infantile fantasies. the multiplicities of promiscuous attachments were repetitions of the abandonments that characterized her developmental experiences and reflected a search for inner regulation.

When the therapist was able to maintain a firm, interpretive framework with clearly defined boundaries, there was room for N to experience the relationship in ways that were determined by the representations of infantile attachments. She then exerted intense pressure to rupture those boundaries, which reflected an intermingling of both healthy and pathological forces. The pressure expressed a pathological search for defensive reinforcement founded upon developmental experiences in which boundaries had not been established but was also motivated by an attempt to gain the experience of containment that facilitated the effectiveness of integrative functions. N's unconscious perception of the qualities she needed, to foster the viability of healthy processes, guided the therapist in abstaining from colluding with her attempts to gain reinforcement of pathological defenses. The therapist's interpretive interventions then aided N in developing perspective and prepared a foundation for replacing the infantile attachments that had controlled her life.

The manner in which an individual engages in the processes of work, play, love, and the activities that sustain them is indicative of the interplay of healthy and pathological forces that are operating within the personality. In M and N, there was a predominance of pathology, with healthy functions periodically evident in response to the unconsciously empathic interpretive interventions of the therapist. In A, there was a predominance of healthy functioning, with the pathological effects of narcissistic structures only minimally present; that was the product of many years of therapeutic involvement.

The course of A's psychotherapy has been presented throughout this volume. It is representative of experiences with a small number of children similarly ravaged during their early development. A's ability to utilize the therapeutic relationship, in fostering the evolution of healthy functioning, seemed to illustrate the qualities in an interaction that facilitate developmental progression.

In the beginning, the therapist was a bridge to the life-sustaining processes that offered hope for A's existence as a functional, autonomous human being. The therapist meant everything to A. A, though important to the therapist, occupied a small segment of the therapist's life. At the end, the bridge was crossed, and A emerged as a feeling, sensitive, functional individual. The therapist no longer meant everything and occupied only a small segment of his life. For the therapist, the lessons learned about himself and about human existence meant everything. The experience with A remains as a light to guide the therapist in all new areas of darkness that are encountered.

References

Balint, E. (1963). On being empty of oneself. *International Journal of Psychoanalysts, 44*, 470–480.

Balint, M. (1968). *The basic fault*. New York: Brunner/Mazel.

Bion, W. R. (1968). *Second thoughts. Selected papers on psychoanalysis*. New York: Basic Books.

Blos, P. (1979). *The adolescent passage*. New York: International Universities Press.

Fairbairn, W. R. D. (1954). *An object-relations theory of the personality*. New York: Basic Books.

Freud, S. (1964). An outline of psychoanalysis. In J. Strachey (Ed. and Trans.), *The standard edition of the complete psychological works of Sigmund Freud* (Vol. 23). London: Hogarth Press. (Original work published 1938)

Grotstein, J. S. (1981). *Splitting and projective identification*. New York: Jason Aronson.

Hartmann, H. (1939). *Ego psychology and the problem of adaptation*. New York: International Universities Press.

Hartmann, H. (1962). Notes on the superego. *The psychoanalytic study of the child* (Vol. 17, pp. 42–81). New York: International Universities Press.

Hoffer, W. (1952). The mutual influences in the development of ego and id. *The psychoanalytic study of the child* (Vol. 7, pp. 31–41). New York: International Universities Press.

Jacobson, E. (1964). The self and the object world. New York: International Universities Press.

Kernberg, O. (1980). *Internal world and external reality*. New York: Jason Aronson Press.

Klein, M. (1955). *New directions in psychoanalysis*. New York: Basic Books.

Kohut, H. (1971). *The analysis of the self*. New York: International Universities Press.

Langs, R. (1977). *The therapeutic interaction: A synthesis*. New York: Jason Aronson.

Mahler, M. S. (1958). Autism and symbiosis. Two extreme disturbances of identity. *International Journal of Psychoanalysis, 39*, 77–83.

Mahler, M. S., Pine F., & Bergman. A. (1975). *The psychological birth of the human infant*. New York: Basic Books.

Mendelsohn, R. (1985). The onset of unconscious perception. *The yearbook of psychoanalysis and psychotherapy* (Vol. 1, pp. 209–239). Hillsdale, NJ: Erlbaum.

Spitz, R. (1955). The primal cavity: A contribution to the genesis of perception and its role for psychoanalytic theory. *The psychoanalytic study of the child* (Vol. 10, pp 215–240). New York: International Universities Press.

Winnicott, D. (1958). Collected papers. New York: Basic Books.

Index